The Wheelchair Evaluation

A CLINICIAN'S GUIDE

Mitchell Batavia, PhD, PT

Associate Professor

Department of Physical Therapy
Steinhardt School of Culture, Education,
and Human Development

New York University

JONES AND BARTLETT PUBLISHERS

Sudbury, Massachusetts

BOSTON   TORONTO   LONDON   SINGAPORE

World Headquarters

Jones and Bartlett Publishers
40 Tall Pine Drive
Sudbury, MA 01776
978-443-5000
info@jbpub.com
www.jbpub.com

Jones and Bartlett Publishers
Canada
6339 Ormindale Way
Mississauga, Ontario L5V 1J2
Canada

Jones and Bartlett Publishers
International
Barb House, Barb Mews
London W6 7PA
United Kingdom

Jones and Bartlett's books and products are available through most bookstores and online booksellers. To contact Jones and Bartlett Publishers directly, call 800-832-0034, fax 978-443-8000, or visit our website www.jbpub.com.

Substantial discounts on bulk quantities of Jones and Bartlett's publications are available to corporations, professional associations, and other qualified organizations. For details and specific discount information, contact the special sales department at Jones and Bartlett via the above contact information or send an email to specialsales@jbpub.com.

The authors, editor, and publisher have made every effort to provide accurate information. However, they are not responsible for errors, omissions, or for any outcomes related to the use of the contents of this book and take no responsibility for the use of the products and procedures described. Treatments and side effects described in this book may not be applicable to all people; likewise, some people may require a dose or experience a side effect that is not described herein. Drugs and medical devices are discussed that may have limited availability controlled by the Food and Drug Administration (FDA) for use only in a research study or clinical trial. Research, clinical practice, and government regulations often change the accepted standard in this field. When consideration is being given to use of any drug in the clinical setting, the health care provider or reader is responsible for determining FDA status of the drug, reading the package insert, and reviewing prescribing information for the most up-to-date recommendations on dose, precautions, and contraindications, and determining the appropriate usage for the product. This is especially important in the case of drugs that are new or seldom used.

Production Credits
Publisher: David Cella
Associate Editor: Maro Gartside
Editorial Assistant: Catie Heverling
Production Director: Amy Rose
Production Assistant: Julia Waugaman
Senior Marketing Manager: Sophie Fleck
Manufacturing and Inventory Control Supervisor: Amy Bacus
Composition: Shawn Girsberger
Cover Design: Scott Moden
Cover Image: © Varina and Jay Patel/ShutterStock, Inc.
Printing and Binding: Malloy Incorporated
Cover Printing: Malloy Incorporated

Library of Congress Cataloging-in-Publication Data
Batavia, Mitch, 1959-
 The wheelchair evaluation : a clinician's guide / by Mitchell Batavia. -- 2nd ed.
   p. ; cm.
 Includes bibliographical references and index.
 ISBN-13: 978-0-7637-6172-1 (pbk.)
 ISBN-10: 0-7637-6172-9 (pbk.)
 1. Wheelchairs--Evaluation. 2. Medical history taking. 3. Orthopedic disability evaluation. I. Title.
 [DNLM: 1. Wheelchairs. 2. Body Constitution. 3. Evaluation Studies as Topic. 4. Medical History Taking--methods. WB 320 B3291w 2010]
 RD757.W4B37 2010
 617'.03--dc22
                                    2009011055
6048
Printed in the United States of America
14 13 12 11 10   10 9 8 7 6 5 4 3 2

Dedication

This book is dedicated to two individuals who have made an indelible mark on my personal and professional growth.

H. Gumprecht

J. G. Gianutsos

"Cut once, measure twice."

—Source unknown

Contents

PART III   THE WHEELCHAIR   109

Chapter 5   The Wheelchair: An Introduction 111

Chapter 6   The Mobility Base 125

**Chapter 7   Seating System and
                    Wheelchair Components 153**

Preface

Changes to the *Second Edition*

The chief aim of this *Second Edition* of *The Wheelchair Evaluation* remains the same—to offer a concise and practical approach to prescribing wheelchairs. It has been 10 years since the *First Edition*, and the landscape for mobility devices has changed dramatically. Although technology has made great advances in mobility options to enhance function and quality of life, acquiring funding for devices has, ironically, become more challenging.

To address these challenges, the changes in this *Second Edition* include (1) four new chapters dedicated to funding, documentation, ethics, and fitting; (2) a Medicare algorithm for wheelchair clinical decision making; (3) updated *evidence* for wheelchair prescription; (4) information on American National Standards Institute (ANSI)/Rehabilitation Engineering and Assistive Technology Society of North America (RESNA) Wheelchair Standards, useful when comparison shopping (e.g., wheelchair strength, stability, durability, fire retardance); (5) photographs depicting wheelchair categories; (6) updated contacts/resources/ links with a greater reliance on Web links; (7) suggested strategies for staying current in the mobility field; and (8) a companion CD containing a PowerPoint slide presentation with videos and animation to complement material contained in the text. I hope this book continues to be useful to the busy clinician who needs a prescription guide.

Why This Book Is Useful

The purpose of this book is to provide a *practical and concise approach* for successfully evaluating and recommending a wheelchair for a patient. Although wheelchair evaluation remains a complex and growing area of specialization, little training is provided in professional schools to teach competency in this area. As a result, clinicians learn on the job through trial and error, often with costly mistakes. In a time when third-party payers are cutting back on funding, it is becoming even more critical to conduct competent evaluations and prescribe appropriate, medically justifiable wheelchairs. It is hoped that this manual will be a practical and concise guide for clinicians and students in health fields who work with physically challenged individuals in need of a wheelchair.

This book has several unique features that distinguish it from other books on this topic. First, the book is *organized* to concisely guide the clinician through a logical sequence in the wheelchair prescription process using a real world (in the trenches) rather than an academic (in the classroom) perspective. The clinician is taken through the necessary steps of patient evaluation, choice of wheelchair components, documentation, and finally, funding using a letter of medical necessity. Second, this book emphasizes *history-taking skills*, which are sadly deficient in most wheelchair-related books and journal articles. Taking a comprehensive history can provide a wealth of vital information that can bear on the success or failure of a wheelchair prescription. Third, this book places special emphasis on evaluating *body shape* variation in order to successfully fit or match the patient to the wheelchair. Body shape is an area that is not emphasized in the education of the health professional, and yet has an important impact in the ultimate fit of an individual with equipment. Fourth, the book was designed to be *portable* and is therefore small enough for the clinician to carry around in the hospital, clinic, school, or nursing home. Finally, this book offers a *general approach* to patient evaluation with emphasis on breadth over depth of subject matter because it is usually what the clinician forgets to assess that leads to a poor result. A general approach has been used because so many clinical decisions must be made based on unique patient needs, regardless of that patient's diagnosis. A seating system, for example, will need to accommodate a hip extension contracture in a patient regardless of whether that patient has cerebral palsy or a spinal cord injury.

In a similar light, this book focuses on wheelchair features driven by patient need rather than reviews of specific brand name components offered by manufacturers, because products may later be added or discontinued. Durable medical equipment suppliers and manufacturers can provide clinicians with information about currently produced wheelchair components once the clinician determines the most important features for a patient.

This book provides several unique and practical aids to facilitate wheelchair prescription. The book utilizes a *question–answer format*. Critical questions that arise during a wheelchair evaluation are asked and then succinctly addressed. *Algorithms* are included to facilitate clinical decision making in choosing wheelchair components. *Illustrations* are provided to clarify difficult concepts and to educate and facilitate communication among clinicians, family members, patients, durable medical equipment suppliers, and manufacturers during a clinic visit. A *sample letter of medical necessity* is included to emphasize important information that needs to be communicated in order to successfully acquire funding for a wheelchair. Finally, *exercises* have been included at the end of each chapter to clarify a concept or drive home a point. These exercises can be used to educate a patient and family member in the clinic or student in the classroom. Every effort has been made to simplify the subject matter. Simplification was done in order to demystify the process and help empower health professionals in their clinical decision making. *The ultimate goal is to provide better patient care.*

Much of the information in this book was empirically derived while working with children and adults with developmental disabilities, but effort has been made to apply this evidence to other populations. Subsequently, information derived from other sources, such as journal articles and texts, has been cited to credit, substantiate, or offer a more complete survey of the subject matter. Although solutions to wheelchair problems are suggested throughout the text, final decisions regarding equipment *MUST* be made by the health professionals, patient, and family who consider all variables and safety issues specific to their case.

The reader may get frustrated by the numerous terms used to refer to the same wheelchair component. An example is the *seat belt*, which may also be referred to as a *pelvic belt*, *lap belt*, or even a *positional belt*. Although attempts are being made to standardize the jargon, variability unfortunately still exists in the literature and industry. Therefore, in this book effort has been made to include all terms that may refer to a piece of equipment so the reader can effectively communicate with others who may still be familiar with only one of the terms.

Helping the patient fit well in a wheelchair involves dealing with multiple and complex variables that are frequently *unique* for that individual. As a result, the evaluation process becomes both an art and a science. Much research still needs to be done in this field to determine how to best serve the patient. An example is the sheer number of variables to consider in choosing a pressure-reducing seat cushion for a patient at risk for a pressure ulcer. Getting it right is not always easy. Hopefully this book will help health professionals to focus on critical areas, anticipate problems, and avoid the "quicksand" associated with a poor wheelchair prescription. Because the wheelchair becomes an extension of the individual and a substitute for the lower limbs, it is imperative that equipment complement the individual's needs and the two fit together into a functional and harmonious whole.

How to Use This Book

This book is organized into four parts and several appendices to provide easy access for wheelchair prescription. Part I is an overview of the wheelchair prescription process and provides a summary of a suggested sequence for the evaluation, important issues to consider during the evaluation, and algorithms for selecting wheelchair bases and components. For example, if only a specific wheelchair part needs to be ordered, the clinician can first refer to the algorithm for component selection and then go to Chapter 7 for more detailed information for that part feature.

In Part II, Chapter 2 addresses history taking (including home accessibility), Chapter 3 covers clinical examination (including measuring a patient for a wheelchair), and Chapter 4 reviews functional examination relevant to manual and power wheelchair prescription. Predictors for power wheelchair performance and the importance of rear wheel position for efficient manual wheelchair use are both underscored in Chapter 4.

In Part III, Chapter 5 is a basic introduction to the wheelchair and discusses general indications, risks, and contraindications for prescription. Issues surrounding wheelchair-related deaths and repetitive strain injuries to the upper extremity are highlighted. Also reviewed are the American National Standards Institute (ANSI)/Rehabilitation Engineering and Assistive Technology Society of North America (RESNA) Wheelchair Standards that may be useful when shopping for wheelchairs. Chapters 6 and 7 cover wheelchair bases (frames) and components (parts), respectively, along with details on features, advantages, disadvantages, and relevant published studies for each piece of equipment.

Part IV includes issues related to ethics (Chapter 8), funding (Chapter 9), documentation and letter writing (Chapter 10), and fittings/dispensing wheelchairs (Chapter 11).

Finally, five appendices include Medicare's algorithm for deciding on mobility assistive equipment (Appendix A), a generic wheelchair evaluation form (Appendix B), resources and links to manufacturers and wheelchair-related topics (Appendix C), a list of differential diagnoses of common wheelchair problems (Appendix D), and body shape considerations (Appendix E). Exercises are included for review at the ends of chapters, which may be particularly useful in the classroom.

A CD complements the textbook to illustrate key concepts in wheelchair prescription using bulleted text, animation, and video clips.

Acknowledgments

Acknowledgments for *Second Edition*

It's been gratifying to revisit and help transport *The Wheelchair Evaluation* into the new millennium. I wish to thank Jones and Bartlett Publishers and David D. Cella, Publisher, for giving the new edition a good home, Maro Gartside, Associate Editor, for assisting with the preparations and copyright issues during the early phases of the manuscript, Catie Heverling, Editorial Assistant, for helping to launch the book and CD into production, and Julia Waugaman, Production Assistant, for shaping the *Second Edition* into final form.

Acknowledgments for *First Edition*

I express my appreciation to Barbara Murphy and Jana Friedman of Butterworth-Heinemann for their support of this project and for the reviewers for their helpful comments. I express my appreciation to Suzanne Schry, director of OT/PT at Terence Cardinal Cooke Health Care Center, for her support in my professional growth and Dr. Moran at NYU for his feedback on ethics. Finally, I acknowledge the durable medical equipment suppliers who have contributed to my skill set, and the patients, who have taught me the most.

About the Author

Dr. Mitchell Batavia is an Associate Professor in the Department of Physical Therapy at New York University. He earned a BS in Physical Therapy from the University of Delaware in 1981, an MA in Motor Learning from Columbia University in 1986, and a PhD in Pathokinesiology/Physical Therapy from New York University in 1997. He completed a Robert Salant post doctoral fellowship at NYU in 1998 and a professional training program in the Feldenkrais Method (Toronto) in 1987. In 2008, Dr. Batavia earned a Postgraduate Diploma in Epidemiology from the Uni- 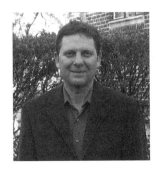 versity of London. In addition to peer-reviewed journal publications in the area of instrument development, augmented feedback, and wheelchair prescription, Dr. Batavia has published three other textbooks, including the *First Edition* of *The Wheelchair Evaluation: A Practical Guide* in 1998 (of which a Korean translation was published in 2004), *Clinical Research for Health Professionals: A User-Friendly Guide* in 2001, and *Contraindications in Physical Rehabilitation: Doing No Harm* in 2006.

Dr. Mitchell Batavia currently teaches wheelchair prescription at NYU.

PART I

Introduction and Overview

CHAPTER 1

Overview

A successful wheelchair fit requires matching an individual's needs with his or her environment (Table 1-1). Consider the following five areas when evaluating an individual for a wheelchair: (1) patient history, (2) clinical impairments, (3) functional abilities, (4) the unique body shape of the patient, and (5) any existing wheelchair. Then consider the patient's environment, both physical (access to home, school, work, buses, and so forth) and social (family, caregiver support). These considerations will provide the clinician with a working hypothesis as to what type of wheelchair may best suit the patient. This working hypothesis should then be tested prior to ordering a wheelchair. The test can come in the form of a

Table 1-1 Overview of the Wheelchair Evaluation Process

Individual	Environment
Patient history	The wheelchair
Patient impairments	Mobility base
Patient skills	Seating system
Unique body shape	Physical and social environment

Evaluate (Patient and Environment)
Hypothesis
Trial/simulation
Recommendation and documentation
Funding
Order
Fitting
Dispensing
Follow-up

trial[1] (borrow the wheelchair) or simulation[2] (putting the patient in a similar physical situation) before the wheelchair is ordered.[3]

Once the evaluation is completed and documented, appropriate recommendations concerning the wheelchair need to be made. Frequently, a letter of medical necessity is required to secure funding for the patient. This letter includes findings from the evaluation and compelling reasons why the wheelchair is required based on medical need.

Upon approval, the wheelchair will be ordered by the supplier. Once it is delivered, it must be properly adjusted to the patient (the fitting). Finally, the patient/family is taught how to safely operate and maintain it before it is dispensed. Future follow-up visits may require reinitiation of the wheelchair process to address equipment wear or changing patient needs.

Preliminary Comments

To Clinicians

- *Designate* one spokesperson for the patient (if more than one advocate comes to the clinic).
- *Listen* to the patient and/or patient advocates.

  - Legitimate requests should be explored.
  - Unjustifiable requests require patient or family education.
  - Use a translator if the patient's language is different from yours and effective communication is doubtful.

- *Safety concerns* must be addressed on the day of the clinic (e.g., sharp hardware that is cutting into the patient should be at least temporarily padded).
- *Teach* proper positioning of the patient and safe use of the wheelchair.

Instructions for the Patient and Caregivers

- Bring a list of all problems or issues concerning the wheelchair to the clinic. A list will ensure that all concerns are mentioned on the day of the clinic.
- Bring in *all* wheelchair components and related equipment on the day of the clinic (including body jackets, braces, typical clothing, or any parts that may have fallen off the wheelchair).
- Have the patient and caregiver provide information to the clinic (e.g., letters, notes, phone numbers) from schools, facilities, therapists, or others involved with the patient's care.
- Inform the patient and caregiver that wheelchairs require medical justification[2] and are therefore based on the particular medical needs of the patient.
- Explain that wheelchairs move and tend to vibrate, so parts on the wheelchair may loosen with time. The wheelchair should be periodically checked

for loose parts, which should be tightened as necessary. If a part falls off the wheelchair and the family is unsure how to properly attach it, request that the family put the part in a bag or box with the patient's name on it so the part does not get lost. Then have the family come to the clinic to have the part reattached as soon as possible.

Working with Suppliers of Durable Medical Equipment

New products come out annually. It's difficult to keep up with the latest technology and new products. That's the supplier's job. Often credentialed as Certified Rehabilitation Technology Suppliers (CRTSs) or Assistive Technology Suppliers (ATSs), these individuals attend annual trade shows so they can learn what's new in the world of durable wheelchair equipment to serve the patients better. Clinicians, patients/family, and caregivers should therefore inform the supplier regarding the patient's needs.[3] They can then research any new and existing products to address those needs.

Selecting a Supplier

Questions to ask:[4]

- What type of patients have you worked with? How long have you been working as a supplier?
- Have you worked with patients in need of custom molded seating systems?
- What line of products do you supply? Which products don't you supply?
- Is your company available for emergencies; do you offer temporary wheelchairs if safety issues arise?
- Can some wheelchair adjustments be done at the clinic? Can you work with tools?
- Do you work with Medicare clients? If so,

    - Are you enrolled as a Medicare supplier?
    - Do you accept assignment?

- Do you hold any certifications?[5]

    - Certified Rehabilitation Technology Supplier (CRTS), credentialed by the National Registry of Rehabilitation Technology Suppliers (NRRTS): www.nrrts.org
    - Assistive Technology Supplier (ATS), credentialed by the Rehabilitation Engineering and Assistive Technology Society of North America (RESNA): www.RESNA.org
    - If a member of the NRRTS, determine whether any complaints have been registered against the supplier/company.

Suggested Sequence of Evaluation

A suggested sequence is included to minimize the amount of patient handling and lifts required during an evaluation (Table 1-2). First take a history, evaluate patient fit and skills, and determine any clinical impairments while the patient sits in the existing wheelchair. Then observe the patient's functional ability while in the wheelchair and during transfers to a mat. The supplier can then inspect the condition of the existing wheelchair while the clinician can continue evaluating the patient on the mat. Finally, the patient can return to sitting for evaluation in a trial wheelchair or in a simulator.

Overview of Patient Examination

The patient examination consists of the patient's problem, past medical history (including systems review), social history, and tests and measures. A very brief outline of these areas follows. For detailed information, refer to Chapter 2 (Patient History), Chapter 3 (Clinical Examination), and Chapter 4 (Functional Examination) in Part II of this book.

Funding Source

As a practical matter, funding agencies should be identified early because they may place limits on a patient's equipment choices.

Chief Complaint

What does the patient say the problem is?

Table 1-2 Suggested Sequence of an Evaluation

Evaluation	Patient Position
History	Sitting
Evaluate fit in existing wheelchair	Sitting
Clinical examination (initial)	Sitting
Functional examination	Sitting and transferring to mat
Clinical examination (continued)	On mat
Passive range of motion, anthropometric, skin, and sensation	
Evaluate condition of existing wheelchair	When patient is out of wheelchair
Trial/Simulation	In trial wheelchair or simulation

List Problems

List problems in order of importance. It may be helpful to offer patients a questionnaire to fill out prior to the clinic visit.[6]

Successes and Failures

Avoid what didn't work in previous prescriptions.

Past Medical History

- *Diagnosis*—The patient's diagnosis informs the clinician about the category of wheelchairs to consider in a prescription. For example, a person with C5 tetraplegia might suggest a power chair, perhaps with a chin control. The diagnosis also offers clues about the medical necessity of equipment. For C5 tetraplegia, tilt-in-space and a pressure-relieving cushion may be considered a medical necessity based on the increased risk for pressure ulcers in this population.
- *Age*—Children need adjustable components to accommodate future growth.[2]
- *Activity level (lifestyle)*—Highly active manual wheelchair users need durable ultralight chairs.
- *Gender*—The center of gravity and fat distribution differ between men and women and may require different postural support.[7]
- *Height*—Tall and short patients may need high and low seat level heights, respectively.[8,9]
- *Weight*—Weight increases the chair's rolling resistance; for obesity, consider the chair's weight capacity.[10]
- *Prognosis*—Prognosis informs the clinician and funding agency as to how long the equipment will be needed. Should the patient rent or purchase? Plan ahead for progressive disorders.[1,11]
- *Precautions*—Are there weight-bearing (skin, bone), range of motion, or exertion restrictions?[11]
- *Surgeries*—Orthopedic surgeries may alter anthropometrics and postural needs.
- *Physical rehabilitation*—Gains made in therapy may reduce future equipment needs.
- *Medication*—Drowsiness due to medications may make power mobility unsafe.[12]
- *Orthotics*—Additional seat space in the wheelchair may be required.
- *Systems review*—For thoroughness, do a chart review of major organ systems.

Social History

- *Residence*—Consider wheelchair accessibility (especially stairs; 32-inch clearance required for doorways; 36 inches for corridors).[13]

- *Caregivers*—Consider the level of support available to maintain equipment (i.e., power mobility, batteries, pneumatic tires).
- *Indoor/outdoor use*—Consider durable frames, shock absorption features, and appropriate power mobility needs for outdoor/rough terrain use.
- *Table surface requirements for work/school/eating*—Determine appropriate armrest style (i.e., desk-type armrests for access to tables; full-length armrests for upper extremity [UE] activities using a lap board).
- *Travel*—Consider a lightweight folding wheelchair for car transportation/ storage, a tie-down feature (certified transit wheelchairs) for bus travel,[14] and nonspill batteries on power mobility for air travel.[15]
- *Hours sitting*—Sitting for extended periods of time (i.e., up time) may require a cushion with greater pressure reduction properties or a tilt/recline wheelchair feature.[16]
- *Age of existing wheelchair*—Wheelchair age determines warrantee status and next funding cycle (often a 5-year period for a new wheelchair).

Tests and Measures: Clinical Examination

- *Anthropometric measurements*—To determine frame size, measure the patient's seat depth, seat width, back height, and heel to knee distances.[17]
- *Postural alignment*—If severe fixed asymmetrical deformities of the trunk or pelvis are present, custom molded postural inserts may be required.[3,18]
- *Active movement*—If no movement/weight shifting ability is possible, consider a good pressure-reducing cushion. If the patient self-propels, consider a manual wheelchair. If not, consider a power wheelchair. For uncontrolled movement, pad/protect from injury.
- *Sitting balance*—Consider lateral and anterior trunk supports if balance is poor, or a reclining or backward tilt-in-space wheelchair to decrease reliance on anterior trunk supports.
- *Primitive reflexes*—Block movements that trigger undesirable reflex activity.
- *Tone*—Extensor tone requires adequate pelvic stabilization. Spasticity may require positioning to reduce tone and foot straps to maintain feet on footrests. Low tone may require reclining/backward tilt-in-space wheelchairs to discourage trunk collapse.
- *Passive range of motion*—Determine whether the patient has sufficient lower extremity (LE) range of motion (ROM) (e.g., 90-degree hip flexion) to fit into a standard wheelchair[3] and UE ROM to reach handrims.
- *Skin*—Determine pressure ulcer risk.
- *Sensation*—If the patient is insensate, a pressure-reducing cushion may be needed. If vision is diminished, power mobility may be unsafe.[19] Evaluate for UE pain (e.g., repetitive strain injury) in handrim wheelchair users.[20]
- *Endurance*—A lighter weight manual wheelchair or power mobility may be required for patients with limited endurance.
- *Strength*—Is strength sufficient to operate all wheelchair components?

- *Cognition*—For power mobility, cause–effect concepts and problem solving are required.[21,22]
- *Perception and judgment*—Consider wheelchair safety. Right CVA patients with hemi neglect may collide into obstacles on their left side. Adequate spatial perception is critical for power mobility.[23,24]
- *Motivation*—The patient must show compliancy with the wheelchair or funding agencies like Medicare will not fund the equipment.[25]
- *Memory*—Memory is required to perform wheelchair procedures (e.g., transfers) safely.
- *Vital functions*—Orthostatic hypotension can limit tolerance for upright sitting.

Tests and Measures: Functional Examination

- *Locomotion*—Unsafe or nonfunctional ambulation requires self-propulsion of a manual wheelchair. Nonfunctional self-propulsion requires safe power mobility or an attendant-operated wheelchair.
- *Transfers*—Evaluate appropriate seat cushion (e.g., stable), front rigging (e.g., swing away/detachable), and armrests (e.g., adjustable/removable) to facilitate specific transfer requirements.
- *Sitting*—High back support may be needed for patients with decreased trunk control and lower activity level in wheelchairs.[26]
- *UE function*—Evaluate ability to self-propel or operate power mobility switches/controls. Observe if configuration of wheelchair is adequate (e.g., rear wheel or joystick locations).

Funding

Funding sources for a wheelchair can be identified at the public and private level.[27] A combination of sources may also be used to fund a wheelchair.[28]

As a practical matter, consider the patient's funding source and criteria for approvals early on. Medicare, for example, will only consider wheelchair approvals for in-home use; outdoor use requests will not be considered.[29] (Refer to Appendix A for the Medicare algorithm.)

Some funding sources include (also see Chapter 9):

- Medicare
- Medicaid
- Veterans Administration
- Vocational rehabilitation
- Workers' compensation
- IDEA (Individuals with Disabilities Education Act)
- Private insurance
- Charitable institutions
- Out of pocket

Documentation: Letter of Medical Necessity

Eligible funding sources typically require justification for a wheelchair in the form of a letter. This letter is referred to as a *letter of medical necessity*. It can be anything from a simple request for the item or a checklist, to a full-fledged letter in prose with point by point justification for each component (i.e., armrest, casters). Medicare has perhaps the most stringent justification requirements[30] and has set the bar for many other insurance carriers (e.g., Medicaid, managed care) who appear to be following its lead.[31] For details on sample letters and forms, refer to Chapter 10.

Awaiting Approval

When the wheelchair recommendation is made, review the order to make sure it's complete and correct. Get a time frame from the supplier as to how long it will take to get funding and order the equipment. This usually takes longer than you think, and you'll be less frustrated if everyone knows how long it will take ahead of time. Take down the supplier's phone number so you can periodically call to determine the status of the wheelchair order. Record dates when paperwork was completed and mailed so you are aware how long to wait before calling. If too much time passes between the initial evaluation and approval/ordering, it would be wise to check whether the patient's medical status or situation has changed (e.g., growth in children, functional abilities, living situation).

Fitting, Training, and Dispensing

Once the wheelchair has been funded, approved, ordered, and delivered, make sure you got what you originally ordered. Also make sure it is properly fitted to the patient. This is best done at the hospital or clinic where the order originated. Several fittings may be required before the wheelchair is acceptable and ready for dispensing. For details regarding fitting, training, and dispensing, refer to Chapter 11.

- Is the order correct and configured as prescribed (e.g., correct wheel axle placement to improve push performance; correct seat back angles)?
- Is the patient adequately positioning in the new wheelchair?
- Is the patient and/or all caregivers trained in the proper use and operation of the wheelchair?
  - Do they have contact information, warrantees, the manufacturer's manual, as well as any special instructions and follow-up information?
- Can patient and caregivers safely operate the wheelchair, or is more training needed before the equipment is dispensed?

If the original evaluation was good, there should be few or no changes when the wheelchair is delivered. If everyone is satisfied with the wheelchair, teach the patient and caregiver how to safely operate it, have the patient sign for it, and dispense it. If you are not satisfied, do not have the patient sign for it yet. Discuss equipment problems with the supplier and reasonable changes in the wheelchair that will make the final fitting acceptable.

Overview of Wheelchair Selection and Algorithms

Selection of a wheelchair requires choosing the most appropriate features based on the patient's needs. The algorithms provided in this section can assist the busy clinician in prescribing major wheelchair components. Lists are included to help the clinician focus on patient examination areas specific to each wheelchair component. For more in-depth information on wheelchair equipment, refer to Chapters 5 through 7.

Mobility bases have been organized by the patient's propulsion ability and postural/orientation needs, although, in principle, there are myriad ways to classify them. Components of the wheelchair include rear wheels/tires, casters, armrests, front rigging, foot rests, handrims, and wheel locks (Figure 1-1). Postural supports include seat cushions, seat inserts, back inserts, anterior/lateral trunk supports, head supports, lap boards, positioning blocks, straps, and seat belts.

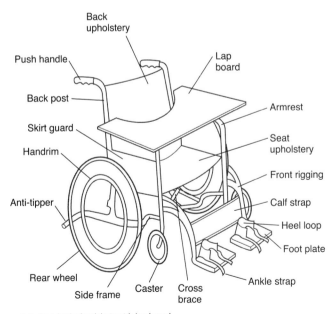

Figure 1-1 Standard wheelchair with lap board

It may be possible to order more than one feature for a particular wheelchair component. For example, an armrest may be adjustable in height, removable, and double length. On the other hand, not all manufacturers offer the same features.

The *key* is to evaluate the patient's needs and then ask the supplier or manufacturer whether the component with the needed features can be ordered and configured with the chair. (Links to manufacturers are provided in Appendix C.)

Mobility Base

The mobility base or frame provides the structure and mobility for the wheelchair. It may be useful to think of types of mobility bases by propulsion ability and body positioning of the patient. Your evaluation will need to be fairly comprehensive to determine a mobility base.

Mobility Bases: Focus of Examination

- ROM of LEs to fit in standard frame
- UE or LE function for wheelchair propulsion
- Posterior stability in wheelchair
- Sitting ability
- Cognition, judgment, perception, and medication
- Muscle tone
- Ability to operate a control switch—for power mobility
- Type of transfer
- Activity level
- Accessibility
- Indoor or outdoor use

Type of Mobility Base (Based on Propulsion Ability)

Determine if the patient is capable of self-propelling a manual wheelchair and how this will be accomplished (i.e., both arms, one arm, feet). If self-propulsion is not feasible, determine if safe power mobility is possible. If only attendant-operated propulsion is possible, determine if the wheelchair will be used solely indoors or both indoors and outdoors (Figure 1-2). Possible mobility bases that address propulsion needs include standard,[11] amputee,[9] ultralight,[32] one-hand drive,[8] hemiplegic,[8] indoor,[8] geriatric wheelchairs,[9] power mobility,[33] power-operated vehicles (scooters),[8] strollers, transport chairs/systems, and lightweight frames.

Type of Mobility Bases (Based on Patient Orientation)

For mobility bases that change patient orientation, determine if the patient is capable of sitting in an upright position, whether gravity-assisted recline or tilt is required due to poor sitting ability and sitting pressure needs, or if a standing orientation is needed for the patient's vocation/avocation (Figure 1-3). Possible choices of mobility bases based on patient orientation include the standard,[11] reclining,[17] tilt-in-space,[34] standing,[35] and elevation frames.[34,35]

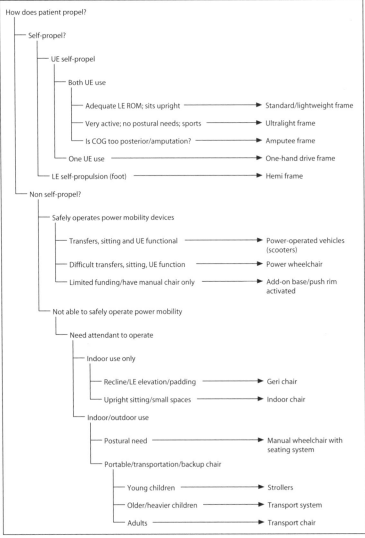

Figure 1-2 Mobility base algorithm based on propulsion ability (UE = upper extremity; LE = lower extremity; ROM = range of motion; COG = center of gravity)

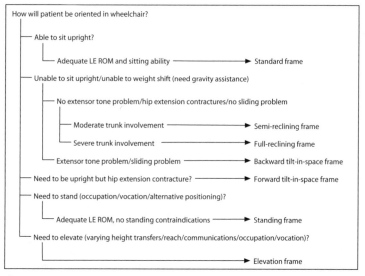

Figure 1-3 Mobility bases algorithm based on orientation need (LE = lower extremity; ROM = range of motion)

Headrests/Supports

Headrests [3,8,34,36] provide midline support for the patient's head if required. Evaluate the patient's ability to maintain midline position of the head. (Make sure head position is not due to inadequate trunk support.) Inspect the shape of the head posteriorly for an occipital ridge area. Ask if the patient travels by public transportation in a wheelchair. Assess safety issues and the ability of caregivers to adequately monitor patients who use equipment around the neck or head (i.e., neck rings, head rings). Head supports may incorporate planar or curved shapes, side panels/pads, neck collars, head rings, and the use of gravity assistance (Figure 1-4).

Headrests/Supports: Focus of Examination

- Head control
- Sitting balance
- Tone/reflexes
- Shape of the head (anthropometrics)
- Use of motor vehicle transportation in wheelchair
- Proper supervision available (i.e., neck rings, head rings)
- Forward sliding activity

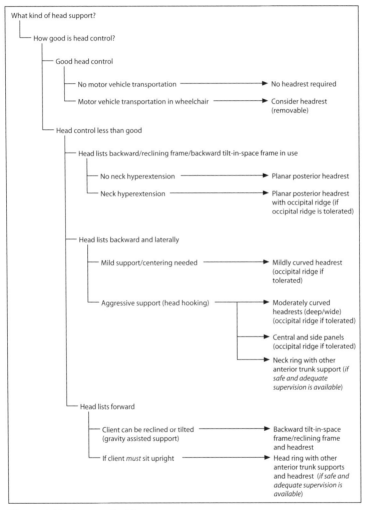

Figure 1-4 Head support algorithm

Back Inserts

Back inserts[3] provide postural support for the patient's trunk and spine. Evaluate the amount of postural support needed to prevent a hammocking effect on the trunk and the amount of contoured back support needed to accommodate a fixed spinal deformity. Determine height requirements of the back insert by assessing the patient's sitting balance and self-propulsion activity level. Back inserts may be planar, curved, or custom molded (Figure 1-5).

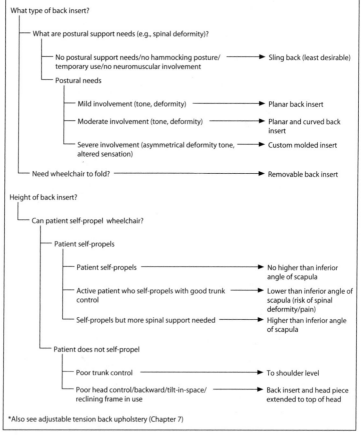

Figure 1-5 Back insert algorithm

Back Inserts: Focus of Examination

- Degree of spinal deformity/need to redistribute pressure
- Trunk control; sitting balance
- Activity level (i.e., sports)
- Tone
- Sensation

Seat Inserts

Seat inserts[37] provide postural support for the pelvis, hips, and lower extremities (thighs). Evaluate the amount of postural support needed to prevent a hammocking effect of the patient's hips and pelvis. Determine the amount of contoured shaping of the seat needed to accommodate deformity and redistribute pressure areas. Seat inserts, like back inserts, may be planar, curved, or custom molded (Figure 1-6).

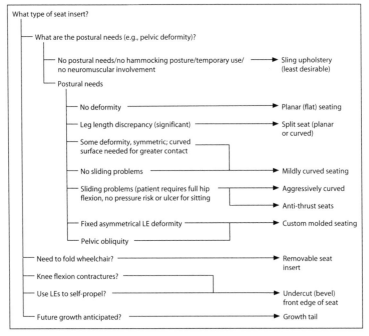

Figure 1-6 Seat insert algorithm (LE = lower extremity)

Seat Inserts: Focus of Examination

- Degree of deformity/need to redistribute pressure
- Leg length discrepancy
- Sliding problems
- Sensation
- Skin integrity and risk factors for pressure ulcers
- Cushion to be used with seat insert

Seat Cushions

Seat cushions[37,38,39] provide comfort and pressure reduction. *No perfect cushion exists for all patients.* Evaluate cushion features (e.g., stability, easy cleaning, light weight, pressure reduction, comfort) that are important for your patient. Note that a protective (incontinence) cover will be needed to protect foam cushions that absorb moisture (i.e., open cell foams). Order two covers so that one can be laundered while the other is in use. Static seat cushions use foam, air, gel, or a combination of these materials. Dynamic seats, on the other hand, use a power source to reduce sitting pressure (Figure 1-7).

Seat Cushions: Focus of Examination

- Incontinence/ease in cleaning cushion
- Weight considerations of cushion
- Caregiver level of support—to maintain and monitor cushion
- Stability for sitting and transfers
- Skin integrity, sensation, and mobility (weight shifting ability)
- Pressure-reducing characteristics of cushion—evaluate individually for each patient
- Risk factors for pressure ulcers

Trunk Supports

Trunk supports[3,9] encourage midline posture and discourage anterior or lateral listing of the trunk. Evaluate if sitting balance or spinal alignment is insufficient anteriorly or laterally. If a harness is considered, assess safety concerns related to straps near the neck area (i.e., risk of strangulation), patient tolerance of straps, and facility policy on restraints. Trunk supports, which include lateral trunk supports, chest straps, chest harnesses, shoulder retractors, and use of gravity (Figure 1-8), should be recommended and used as positioning devices rather than as restraints. Try to use the least restrictive and safest approach to achieve seating goals.

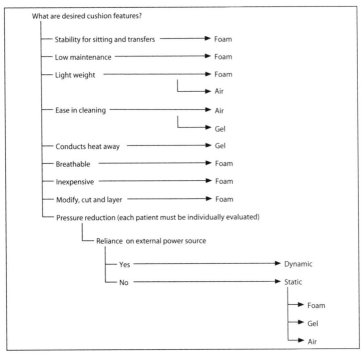

Figure 1-7 Seat cushion algorithm

Trunk Supports: Focus of Examination

- Postural/spinal alignment
- Sitting balance
- Tone/reflexes
- Tactile defensiveness/sensitivity
- Facility policy on restraints
- Safety concerns: harness near neck region

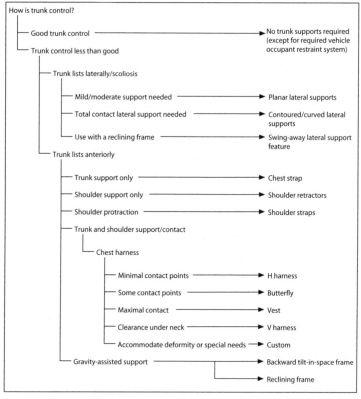

Figure 1-8 Trunk support algorithm

Armrests

Armrests[32,40] provide support for the upper extremities. Determine the type of armrest based on the type of transfers, upper extremity support needs, and requirements for work, school, and eating. Armrest features address armrest length, height adjustability, detachability, durability, and effect on overall wheelchair width (Figure 1-9).

Armrests: Focus of Examination

- Type of transfers
- Amount of UE support needed

- School/work—use of desk or lap board
- Clearance through doorways
- Ability to reach wheels to self-propel
- Use of reclining frame

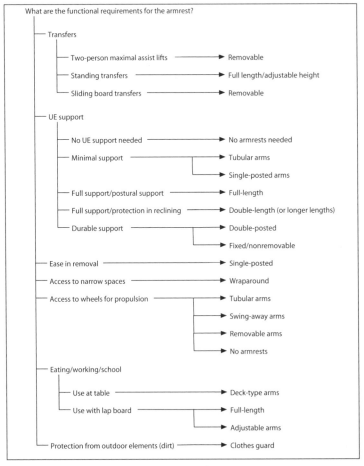

Figure 1-9 Armrest algorithm (UE = upper extremity)

Lap Board

Lap boards[8,11,35,41] rest over the armrests and provide a table surface for the patient while in the wheelchair. Determine if the patient will need a lap board for additional upper extremity support/rest, feeding, programming activities, communication, or power control interfacing. Lap board features include use of solid or clear materials, optional cutout areas for UE clearance to reach rear wheels or for joystick placement, easels and overlays for communication, rims to prevent objects from falling off the edge of the board, and straps to keep the board from sliding off the armrests (Figure 1-10).

Consider the type of hardware used to secure the lap board to the armrest because some mechanisms are more difficult to operate and less reliable in performance than others. Note that lap boards generally require the support of full-length armrests and may tip forward if secured to desk-type armrests. They can also be quite heavy, when customized.

Lap Board: Focus of Examination

- UE edema requiring elevation
- Painful shoulder requiring support
- Table surface for work, school, and play activities
- Surface for communication or feeding
- Perceptual neglect of UE

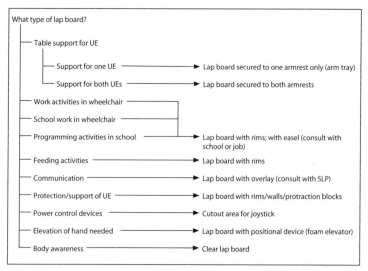

Figure 1-10 Lap board algorithms (UE = upper extremity; SLP = speech language pathologist)

Positioning Blocks and Straps

Positioning blocks and straps may help some patients maintain a more neutral and midline position while in the wheelchair. Evaluate if the patient's extremities are in or out of midline. Positioning blocks include protraction blocks, hip guides, knee adductors, pommels, and knee blocks. Straps and webbing include heel loops and ankle straps (Figure 1-11).

Positioning Blocks/Straps: Focus of Examination

- Asymmetrical postural alignment of UEs and LEs
- Muscle tone and pathological reflexes[42]

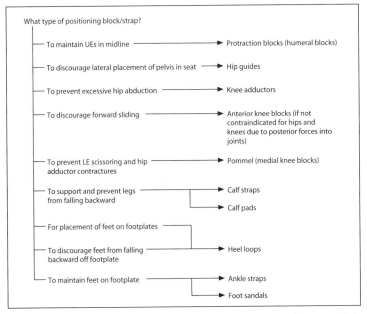

Figure 1-11 Positioning block/straps algorithm (UE = upper extremity; LE = lower extremity)

Wheel Locks (Brakes)

Wheel locks[8] prevent the wheelchair from rolling. Evaluate the patient's motor ability to independently operate wheel locks. Wheel locks may be toggle, level, or scissor in style. Some wheel locks may be mounted high or low based on the patient's level of function and reach (Figure 1-12).

Wheel Locks: Focus of Examination

- UE coordination, strength, and reach
- Hilly terrain

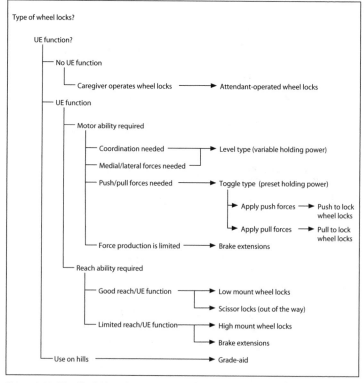

Figure 1-12 Wheel lock algorithm (UE = upper extremity)

Rear Wheels

Rear wheels permit the wheelchair to roll. Rear wheel selection is based on several features such as wheel weight versus durability,[38] angle of the wheels (camber), storage, and position of rear wheels to influence the stability or mobility of the wheelchair. As previously noted, it is possible to request more than one feature for your patient. For example, your patient may need spokeless (molded) wheels that are cambered and have a quick release feature to address durability, lateral stability, and portability requirements (Figure 1-13).

Rear Wheels: Focus of Examination

- Need for propulsion efficiency
- Need for maneuverability
- Need for stability
- Need for storage
- Need for durability
- Need for light weight

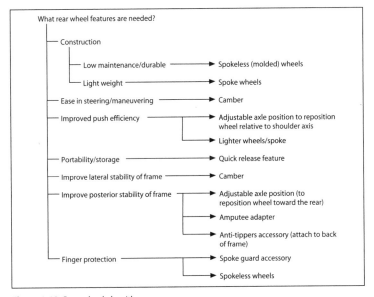

Figure 1-13 Rear wheel algorithm

Rear Tires

Rear tires surround the rear wheels, contact the ground, and transmit forces to and from the wheelchair. Focus the evaluation on whether the wheelchair will be used primarily indoors or outdoors. Three types of tires include solid,[8] pneumatic (air),[1] and airless (filled) (Figure 1-14). If a pneumatic tire is selected, consider ordering an air pump to maintain proper tire pressure level.

Tires: Focus of Examination

- Indoor or outdoor terrain
- Ability to maintain equipment
- Comfortable ride
- Rolling resistance of tire

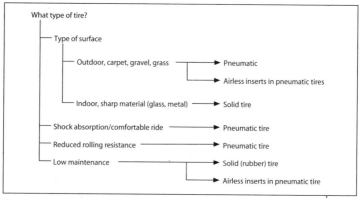

Figure 1-14 Tire algorithm

Handrims

Handrims are mounted onto the rear wheels and are grasped by the patient in order to self-propel the wheelchair. Evaluate handrim diameter according to speed or strength requirements of the patient during self-propulsion. Determine the need for coverings or projections based on the patient's hand function. Choices for handrims include different size diameters,[32,38] and standard rims, coated rims,[32] or rims with projection[38] (Figure 1-15). Consider the use of gloves to reduce the risk of friction burns from handrims when stopping the wheelchair.

Handrims: Focus of Examination

- Hand function and deformity
- Strength of UEs
- Need for speed (e.g., sports)

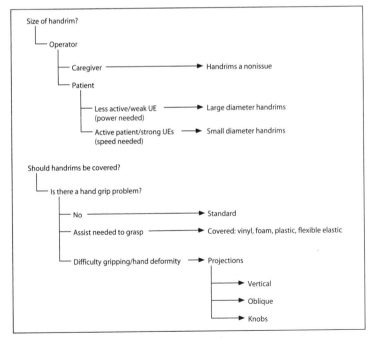

Figure 1-15 Handrim algorithm (UE = upper extremity)

Casters

Casters[40] are small wheels (usually in the front) that enable the wheelchair to turn and change direction. Determine caster size according to caster performance requirements (i.e., shock absorption, maneuverability, negotiation over cracks). Caster sizes range from 2 to 8 inches in diameter (Figure 1-16).

Casters: Focus of Examination

- Need for comfortable ride
- Need for maneuverability/performance
- Surface conditions
- Clearance of front rigging

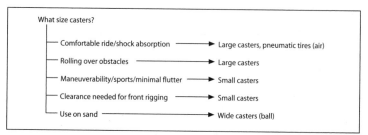

Figure 1-16 Caster algorithm

Seat Belt/Positioning Belt

Seat belts provide safety during transportation. If properly used, they can also be used as positioning belts to help stabilize the patient's pelvis in order to maintain good postural alignment. Focus your evaluation on hand function, posture, muscle tone, and body size. Determine the patient's ability to operate different types of seat belts. The choice of seat belts include Velcro, buckle, airplane, auto, and fastex. Evaluate the need for additional pelvic stabilization by using peroneal straps[36] or a sub-ASIS (anterior superior iliac spine) bar[9] to address strong extensor tone or sliding problems (Figure 1-17). Choose belt size based on body size (Figure 1-18).

Seat Belt/Positioning Belt: Focus of Examination

- Hand function to operate belt
- Anthropometrics (body size)—to determine belt length and width
- Postural support needs at pelvis
- Amount of extensor tone

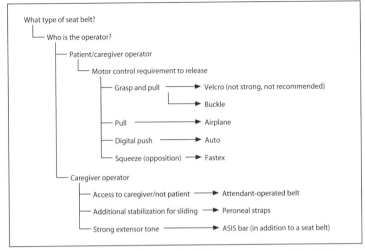

Figure 1-17 Seat belt/positioning belt algorithm (ASIS = anterior superior iliac spine)

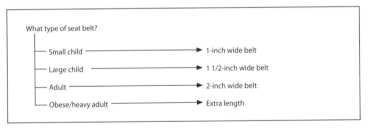

Figure 1-18 Size of belt

Front Rigging

Front rigging provides a support surface for the patient's lower legs and feet. Focus the evaluation on LE range of motion, transfer abilities, and tolerance of dependent LEs. Choice of features,[40] include fixed (with flip-up footplates), swing-away, detachable, or elevating front rigging (Figure 1-19). Patients with bilateral above knee (AK) amputation who are nonambulatory may not need front rigging; other patients, who use their feet to propel, may need front rigging for support only during long distance transportation.

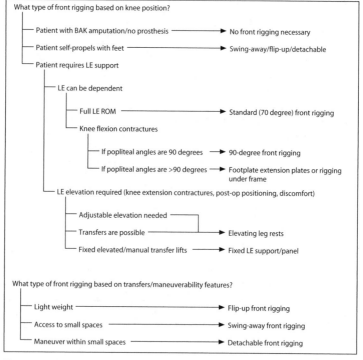

Figure 1-19 Front rigging algorithm (BAK = bilateral above knee; LE = lower extremity; ROM = range of motion)

Front Rigging: Focus of Examination

- Knee ROM limitations (e.g., ankylosis of knee)
- Cast (LE)
- Type of transfer
- Poor tolerance for dependent position
- Environment—small living spaces
- Diagnosis (AK amputation)
- Self-propulsion using LE

Footplates

Footplates provide a flat support surface for the feet. Determine the type of footplate based on the need to support the patient's feet in whatever available ankle range, foot range, and foot location is possible. Focus the evaluation on LE range of motion, body dimensions, and postural symmetry of the LEs. Footplate features include standard, adjustable angle, footplate extenders, one-piece footboards, and a custom footbox (Figure 1-20). Consider a larger size footplate to support large feet and to protect toes if they overhang or if there is the possibility of trauma from bumping into walls.

Footplates: Focus of Examination

- ROM limitations—foot and ankle deformity
- Anthropometrics—leg length discrepancy, foot size
- Posture—LEs windswept

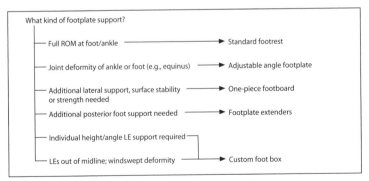

Figure 1-20 Footplate algorithm (ROM = range of motion; LE = lower extremity)

Storage

Finally, think of storage needs for your patient such as utility bags for medication, storage racks for assistive devices and feeding poles, and of course, the storagability of the wheelchair itself (Figure 1-21).

Storage: Focus of Examination

- Ventilator need
- Continuous feeding need
- Continuous (IV) medication need
- Assistive device use
- Significant storage needs (medications, educational, change in clothing, diapers)
- Wheelchair storage/portability

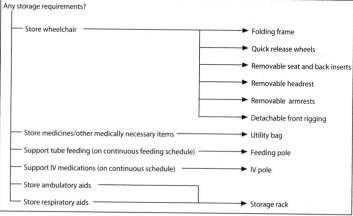

Figure 1-21 Storage algorithm

Exercises

1. Describe nine stages involved in wheelchair prescription.
2. What issue might you discuss with the caregiver or patient over the phone before they attend a clinic for a wheelchair evaluation?
3. List at least 10 different types of wheelchair components that can be prescribed.
4. How might a clinician focus the examination to order each of the following wheelchair components?

    a. Mobility bases
    b. Seat belts
    c. Front rigging
    d. Footplates
    e. Handrims
    f. Rear wheels
    g. Rear tires
    h. Casters
    i. Wheel locks
    j. Armrests
    k. Seat cushions
    l. Seat inserts
    m. Back inserts
    n. Trunk supports
    o. Head supports

5. List some features for each of the following wheelchair components:

    a. Mobility bases
    b. Seat belts
    c. Front rigging
    d. Footplates
    e. Rear wheels
    f. Rear tires
    g. Casters
    h. Handrims
    i. Wheel locks
    j. Armrests
    k. Seat cushions
    l. Seat inserts
    m. Back inserts
    n. Trunk supports
    o. Head supports

OVERVIEW

6. Evaluation form:
   a. How would you design your own wheelchair evaluation form to suit the needs of your clinic?
   b. What major headings would you include?
   c. Develop an evaluation form and then compare yours to the one in Appendix B. (Did you leave anything out or would you include any additional information?)
7. Describe an efficient sequence for conducting a wheelchair evaluation.

References

1. Behrman AL. Clinical perspectives on wheelchair selection: factors in functional assessment. *J Rehabil Res Dev.* 1990;2(Supp):17–27.
2. Freney D. Pediatric seating. *Home Health Care Dealer/Supplier.* 1995;Sept/Oct:103–105.
3. Taylor SJ. Evaluating the client with physical disabilities for wheelchair sitting. *Am J Occup Ther.* 1987;41:711–716.
4. Walls G. Choosing the right cushion. *Rehabil Manage.* 2002;15(1):32–36.
5. Edlich RF, Winters KL, Nelson KP et al. Technological advance in power wheelchairs. *J Long Term Eff Med Implants.* 2004;14(2):107–129.
6. McDonald R, Surtees R, Wirz S. A comparison between parents' and therapists' views of their child's individual seating systems. *Int J Rehabil Res.* 2003;26:235–243.
7. Fay BT, Thorman TA, Cooper R. The yin and yang of wheelchair use. March 2001. Available at: http://www.rehabpub.com/ltrehab/32001/2.asp. Accessed November 4, 2008.
8. Wilson AB, McFarland SR. Types of wheelchairs. *J Rehabil Res Dev.* 1990;2(Supp):104–116.
9. Redford JB. Seating and wheeled mobility in the disabled elderly population. *Arch Phys Med Rehabil.* 1993;74:877-885.
10. Mercer JL, Boninger M, Koontz A, Ren D, Dyson-Hudson T, Cooper R. Shoulder joint kinetics and pathology in manual wheelchair users. *Clin Biomech.* 2006;21(8):781–789.
11. Mattingly D. Wheelchair selection. *Orthop Nurs.* 1993;12:11–17.
12. Eddy L. *Physical Therapy Pharmacology.* St. Louis, MO: Mosby Year Book; 1992:107–115.
13. American National Standards Institute. *American National Standard for Buildings and Facilities: Providing Accessibility and Usability for Physically Handicapped People. Accessible Elements and Spaces (A117.1).* New York: American National Standards Institute; 1986:16–73.
14. School bus transportation of children with special health care. Committee on Injury and Poison Prevention. *Pediatr.* 2001;108:516–518.
15. Southwest Airlines. Traveling tips for customers with disabilities: manual and power wheelchairs. Available at: http://www.southwest.com/travel_center/disability.html#wheelchairs. Accessed November 4, 2008.
16. Hobson DA. Comparative effects of posture on pressure and shear at the body-seat interface. *J Rehabil Res Dev.* 1992;29(4):21–31.
17. Delisa JA, Greenberg S. Wheelchair prescription guidelines. *Am Fam Physician.* 1982;24:145–150.

18. Grunewald J. Wheelchair selection from a nursing perspective. *Rehabil Nurs.* 1986;11:31–32.

19. Batavia M. *Contraindications in Physical Rehabilitation.* St Louis, MO: Saunders; 2006.

20. Curtis KA, Drysdale GA, Lanza RD, Kolber M, Vitolo RS, West R. Shoulder pain in wheelchair users with tetraplegia and paraplegia. *Arch Phys Med Rehabil.* 1999;80(4):453–457.

21. Rosenblith JF, Sims-Knight JE. *In the Beginning: Development in the First Two Years.* Newbury Park, CA: Sage; 1989:411–415.

22. Furumasu J, Guerette P, Tefft D. Relevance of the pediatric powered wheelchair screening test for children with cerebral palsy. *Dev Med & Child Neurol.* 2004;46:468–474.

23. Siev E, Freishtat B, Zoltan B. *Perceptual and Cognitive Dysfunction in the Adult Stroke Patient: A Manual for Evaluation and Treatment.* Rev ed. Thorofare, NJ: Slack; 1986:53–87.

24. Webster JS, Rapport LJ, Godlewski MC, Abadee PS. Effect of attentional bias to right space on wheelchair mobility. *J Clin Exp Neuropsychol.* 1994;16(1):129–137.

25. Centers for Medicare and Medicaid Services. An algorithmic approach to determine if mobility assistive equipment is reasonable and necessary for medicare beneficiaries with a personal mobility deficit (CR3791—Mobility Assistive Equipment (MAE)). *MLN Matters.* 2005, June 3; MM3791. Available at: http://www.cms.hhs.gov/MLNMatters Articles/downloads/MM3791.pdf. Accessed January 15, 2008.

26. Kamenetz HL. *The Wheelchair Book: Mobility for the Disabled.* Springfield, CT: CC Thomas;1969:132–134.

27. Buning ME, Schmeler MR, Crane B. Funding for wheelchairs in general. Available at: http://www.wheelchairnet.org/WCN_ProdServ/Funding/funding.html. Accessed January 26, 2009.

28. Guerette P, Tefft D, Furumasu J. Pediatric powered wheelchairs: results of a national survey of providers. *Asst Technol.* 2005;17:144–158.

29. Medicare Rights Center. Forcing isolation: Medicare's "in the home" coverage standard for wheelchairs. *Care Manage J.* 2005;6(1):29–37.

30. Centers for Medicare and Medicaid Services. Overview of Medicare coverage of power mobility devices (PMD): power wheelchairs and power operated vehicles (POVs). May 2007. ICN 00626. Available at: http://www.cms.hhs.gov/MLNProducts/downloads/PMDBrochure07_Quark11.pdf. Accessed November 4, 2008.

31. Dicianno BE, Tovey E. Power mobility device provision: understanding Medicare guidelines and advocating for clients. *Arch Phys Med Rehabil.* 2007;88:807–816.

32. Ragnarsson KT. Clinical perspectives on wheelchair selection: prescription considerations and a comparison of conventional and light weight wheelchairs. *J Rehabil Res Dev.* 1990;2(Supp)8–16.

33. Miles-Tapping C, MacDonald LJ. Lifestyle implications of power mobility. *Phys and Occup Ther Geriatr.* 1994;12:31–49.

34. Harrymann SE, Warren LR. Positioning and power mobility. In Church G, Glennen S, eds. *The Handbook of Assistive Technologies.* San Diego: Singular; 1992:55–92.

35. Warren CG. Technical considerations: power mobility and its implications. *J Rehabil Res Dev.* 1990;2(Supp):74–85.

36. Bergen AF, Presperin J, Tallman T. *Positioning for Function: Wheelchairs and Other Assistive Technologies.* Valhalla, NY: Valhalla Rehabilitation; 1990:13–62.

37. Garber SL. Classification of wheelchair cushions. *Am J Occup Ther.* 1979;10:652–654.

38. Currie DM, Hardwick K, Marburger RA, Britell CW. Wheelchair prescription and adaptive seating. In Delisa JL, Gans BM, eds. *Rehabilitation Medicine: Principles and Practice,* 2nd ed. Philadelphia: JB Lippincott; 1993:563–585.

OVERVIEW

roman36 Chapter 1: Overview

39. Garber SL. Wheelchair cushions: a historical review. *Am J Occup Ther.* 1985;39:453–459.
40. Kohlmeyer KM, Stevens S, Ueberfluss J. Wheelchairs. In Yarkony GM, ed. *Spinal Cord Injury: Medical Management and Rehabilitation.* Gaithersburg, MD: Aspen; 1994:169–172.
41. Brant J. Wheelchair clinics work. *Occup Ther Health Care.* 1988;5:67–70.
42. Fiorentino MR. *Reflex Testing Methods for Evaluating CNS Development.* Springfield, IL: Charles C Thomas; 1981:14–21.

PART II

The Individual

CHAPTER 2

Patient History

What's the patient's story? Past and present patient problems will provide information on what the patient may need in the future. Taking a history requires active listening skills.

Source

Designate a Spokesperson for the Patient

Avoid a room full of people screaming to be heard. Instead, designate one spokesperson to provide relevant patient information. This may be the patient, the legal guardian, or a family member. Other reliable persons can be interviewed later.

Who Should That Spokesperson Be?

The key is to talk to the person who spends the *most time* with the patient and therefore is familiar with the patient's lifestyle and behaviors. This may, of course, be the patient. If, however, the patient cannot communicate, then the contact person may be a family member, longtime friend, home health aide, or even housekeeper. Get the story from the right person.

Chief Complaint

What Brought You to the Clinic Today?

What's the chief problem? In other words, what motivated the patient or family to come for help? Write down this information. It not only will give the patient the feeling that someone is listening, but also will help to focus on problems *important to the patient.*

Problem List

List Problems with the Existing Wheelchair

Make a list of all patient and family concerns. Don't leave until all concerns are aired. Any injury-related concerns need to be addressed on the day of the clinic.

Here are some of the more common wheelchair problems (also see Appendix D):

- Wheelchair is too small (outgrown)
- Wheelchair is "falling apart" (old)
- Patient is developing a pressure ulcer
- Wheelchair is difficult to push
- Wheelchair tips over
- Patient slides out of wheelchair
- Patient is "uncomfortable" in wheelchair
- Head falls forward in the wheelchair
- Patient falls (listing) to the side
- Patient "hooks" head around the headrest
- Patient is injuring self in the wheelchair
- Patient is sitting slumped in wheelchair
- Wheel locks (brakes) are broken
- Wheelchair does not fold

Daily Family Concerns

Clinicians should consider issues from the perspective of the family. In an interesting qualitative study that compared parent and therapist perspectives on children's seating systems, McDonald et al. noted that parents were more concerned about practical day-to-day management issues (transfers, socialization, weight of the device, car storage) whereas therapists were more focused on technical aspects (posture, accessing switches).[1]

Prioritize What's Important to the Patient

Just because a clinician uncovered a problem, doesn't mean the patient's concerns were addressed in the clinic that day. Using a car repair analogy, you can bring your car to a mechanic with a noisy transmission problem, have a broken car door fixed, and still leave with a noisy transmission. Make sure the patient's chief concern is addressed on the day of the clinic.

Successes and Failures

What things have worked and failed in the past and presently? Does the patient or family have any suggestions for successful future modifications? There's no point in recommending something that's been previously tried and failed. If the patient has a new idea, hear him or her out. Patients and family members frequently have innovative and creative solutions to a problem. I once met a father who solved a front rigging problem on his daughter's wheelchair using plumbing pipe supplies.

Past Medical History

Next, familiarize yourself with the patient's medical background, because it will offer cues to the prescription.

Demographics

Age

For children, anticipate growth needs when ordering a wheelchair. The average seating system will sustain 2 to 3 years of child growth before a new seating system is needed.[2] For elders, consider the impact of comorbidities that may affect safety and comfort: judgment, vision, circulation (ulcer risks), and back deformities (e.g., dowager's hump)[3] in need of accommodation.

Gender

Men and women may differ in terms of body fat distribution, limb length, and the center of gravity. Comparatively, women have smaller girth and shorter linear measurements. These factors, in turn, may affect wheelchair fit such as reaching the handrims. Female manual wheelchair users also differ in biomechanical aspects of manual propulsion from their male counterparts, producing less pushrim forces and requiring more frequent push cycles.[4] (Also see Appendix E.) Furthermore, there is some evidence that female manual wheelchair users may be at a greater risk for shoulder pathology, although the reasons are unclear. In a small study of 14 persons (8 male, 6 female) with paraplegia, who were scanned for shoulder pathology, all of the women but only one man revealed positive MRIs ($P = 0.001$), despite being no different (statistically) in age, spinal cord injury (SCI), onset age, and body mass index (BMI) from the remaining sample.*[5] Finally, women's daily activities differ from men's in some obvious ways with regard to self-care (catheter management), menstrual cycle, reproductive plans, and perhaps baby/child care, all of which can impact on wheelchair needs.[6]

Height

Tall patients may require a higher seat to facilitate transfers and clear feet from dragging on the floor.[7] Short stature patients, on the other hand, may need a lower seat or hemi chair.[7,8] Children's seating can be lower to the floor.

Weight

Heavier patients may exceed the weight capacity that a standard wheelchair frame is warranteed for and may therefore require a heavier duty frame construction. There is also evidence that increased body mass is associated with higher shoulder forces[9] and greater upper extremity (UE) pathology in persons with paraplegia

---

* The sample consisted of persons, mean age 32.8 years, who were 10.4 mean years postinjury and had a SCI injury level of T2 or below.[5]

(i.e., median nerve function, acromioclavicular edema, coracoacromial thickening). It may be that heavier individuals increase the chair's rolling resistance, thereby requiring greater UE forces to propel the chair.[10,11] (Also see Obesity.)

Diagnosis

Knowing the patient's diagnosis can help narrow your choice of wheelchairs. For example, a small premature infant who cannot self-propel a wheelchair may benefit from a stroller (for a few years) with adaptive inserts to provide postural support. A cardiac patient who sits well but has limited endurance may benefit from a power-operated vehicle (scooter). A stroke patient who is paralyzed on one side of his or her body may benefit from a wheelchair with a seat that is low to the floor. The unaffected foot can then reach the floor in order to assist the patient in propelling the wheelchair. A nonambulatory patient with a severe scoliosis may require customized seating that is molded around the contours of the back deformity. Finally, a spinal cord–injured patient who cannot use his or her arms or legs to self-propel can often benefit from a power wheelchair.

Wheelchair recommendations based on some patient diagnoses are listed in the following sections, although much will depend on the extent of involvement. In practice, final recommendations *must* be based on a full evaluation of all factors that can impact a prescription.

Obesity

The obese patient may require a wide, heavy-duty frame with shock absorption features to address body dimensions and weight capacity of the wheelchair. (Also see Weight.) Bariatric wheelchairs (for persons >100 pounds beyond ideal weight)[12] are wider, reinforced, more expensive (double the price of standard frames), and may require wider door access than the 32-inch doorway clearance width specified under Americans with Disabilities Act (ADA) Architectural Barriers Act Accessibility Guidelines.[13]

- Heavy-duty wheelchair (double cross-braced)
- Wide adult/oversized wheelchair (20 inches or wider)
- Extra-long seat belt
- Full-length armrests to assist in transfers[7]
- Shock absorption features such as pneumatic (air) tires[14]

Undernutrition/Starvation

Thin, undernourished patients are at high risk for pressure ulcers[15] and may need padding under straps and belts, and pressure relief under ischia to address the potential for pressure ulcers.

- Pad straps and belts, if used
- Pressure-relieving cushion

Arthrogryposis

The patient with arthrogryposis may need power mobility if UE range of motion restricts self-propulsion abilities. A molded back insert may be required if significant spinal deformity is present.

- Power mobility if upper extremity range is limited
- Custom molded inserts for spinal deformities

Traumatic Brain Injury (Severe)

Depending of the extent of involvement, the nonambulatory patient with a severe brain injury may need postural support to maintain symmetrical posture, address the influence of abnormal tone/reflexes, and prevent contractures such as equinus deformities. The frame may need to be heavy duty if the patient is aggressive and applies excessive forces while in the wheelchair.

- Heavy-duty/strong frame
- Custom postural inserts
- Sufficient foot support to discourage risk of equinus deformity

Cerebral Vascular Accident (CVA)

The patient who had a stroke and has only one functional UE and lower extremity (LE) may need a hemiplegic or one-hand drive frame to self-propel. A brake extension on the involved side can facilitate reach to wheel locks. A lap board or support surface can help elevate an edematous hand, protect and enhance awareness of a neglected UE, and support (but not reduce) a painful subluxed shoulder. Right CVA patients who present with hemi neglect may need further evaluation because they may tend to run into objects to the left and directly in front of their wheelchair path.[16]

- Hemiplegia wheelchair
- One-hand/arm drive mechanism or frame
- Lap board
- Brake extension

Rheumatoid Arthritis

The rheumatoid arthritic patient may benefit from a high seat to facilitate transfers, postural support to rest involved body parts, large wheels to facilitate self-propulsion, and brake extensions to facilitate reach of wheel locks.[17]

- Higher seat
- Large rear wheels
- Elevating/removable leg rests if LE involvement
- Brake extensions
- Neck support piece if cervical involvement

Bilateral Lower Extremity Amputee

The patient with an amputation may need an amputee frame or an amputee adapter kit to improve posterior stability and prevent backward tipping of the wheelchair because these patients, having lost anterior mass, will have a more posteriorly displaced center of gravity. In addition, the residual limb lengths may be different and therefore require separate amounts of support on each side of the seat (i.e., split seat) for proper positioning.

- Amputee wheelchair
- Amputee adapter
- Split seat insert (for below knee [BK] amputee)
- No front rigging[18] (if bilateral [AK] patient is nonambulatory and has no prostheses)

SCI: Tetraplegia

Depending on the level of injury, patients with tetraplegia will need a pressure-relieving cushion, a lightweight frame with an adjustable axle if self-propulsion is possible, or a power wheelchair with power tilt/recline features and a back-up manual wheelchair if the SCI level is high (e.g., C4). A pushrim-activated, power-assisted wheelchair (PAPAW) may be an alternative for some patients with limited UE function.[19]

C1–C4 Tetraplegia[20]

- Power wheelchair
- Pressure-relieving cushion
- Powered recline or tilt mechanism
- Back-up manual wheelchair[21]
- Life support system (respirator) mounting[22]

C5 Tetraplegia

- Power wheelchair with hand controls
- Back-up manual wheelchair[21]
- Pressure-reducing cushion
- Manual wheelchair with oblique handrim projections

C6 Tetraplegia

- Lightweight/ultralightweight manual wheelchair, adjustable axle, gloves, coated handrims, projections
- Power wheelchair (for long distance lifestyle needs)
- Pressure-reducing cushion

C7–C8 Tetraplegia

- Lightweight/ultralightweight manual wheelchair, adjustable axle
- Pressure-reducing cushion

SCI: Paraplegia

The person with paraplegia needs a pressure-reducing cushion and a lightweight or ultralightweight wheelchair (preferably) to facilitate self-propulsion.

- Lightweight/ultralightweight manual wheelchair with adjustable axle
- Pressure-reducing cushion
- Gloves to prevent friction burns from handrims

Triplegia

The triplegic patient with only one functional UE may need a one-hand drive frame if hand function is adequate. Postural alignment should be monitored because there is a tendency to lean to the side and out of midline to operate one-hand drive mechanisms.[22]

- One-hand drive manual wheelchair; power mobility may be an alternative.

Myelomeningocele

The myelomeningocele patient may need a molded back or pressure relief area to accommodate spinal deformity. A pressure-reducing cushion can address a pressure ulcer risk due to lack of sensation. An accommodating head support may be needed if hydrocephalus is present and head control is poor. Be aware that persons with spina bifida may be allergic to latex, which is commonly found in wheelchair parts such as tires.

- Manual wheelchair with growth capability
- Back insert with pressure relief for myelomeningocele
- Head support for hydrocephalus, if needed
- Pressure-reducing cushion
- Incontinence seat covers

Fixed Scoliosis (Severe)

The nonambulatory patient with a severe scoliosis may need a custom molded back insert to accommodate spinal deformity.

- Custom molded back insert

Hip Dislocation with Fixed Windswept Deformity

The patient with a hip dislocation and an asymmetrical windswept deformity may take up space in the wheelchair due to asymmetrical sitting. The pelvis may be oblique and LEs will both deviate to the same side. A wider frame (to accommodate the windswept position) and a pressure-reducing cushion or molded seat (to redistribute excessive weight bearing under the involved hip joint) may be required.

- Wider frame
- Pressure-reducing cushion or custom molded seat

Cardiac Patient

Cardiac patients may need a power mobility device if there are exertion restrictions or endurance is severely compromised.

- Power-operated vehicle (scooter)
- Power wheelchair

Self-Abusive/Agitated Patients

The self-abusive patient may need a stable, heavy-duty frame with padding on hard surfaces for safety and nondetachable equipment so that components do not become projectiles.

- Nondetachable components (arms, front riggers, brake extensions)
- Heavy-duty frame (if strong body activity)
- Padded hard surfaces to reduce risk of injuring patient
- Anti-tippers (if body rocking)

Seizure Disorder

The seizure patient may require padding on hard surfaces that may cause injury from impact during a seizure. Power mobility may be unsafe.

- Pad wheelchair components to reduce risk of injuring patient

Total Hip Arthroplasty

The patient with a total hip replacement may need a high seat level to discourage excessive hip flexion during transfer activities during the postoperative recovery period. A pommel may help to prevent hip adduction if necessary.[23]

- Firm, thick cushion, to transfer without leaning forward or increasing hip flexion
- Pommel

Geriatric Patient

The geriatric patient may need full-length adjustable armrests to facilitate transfers, a seat cushion to provide comfort or pressure reduction, a curved back support to accommodate any fixed kyphotic spinal deformity (e.g., dowager hump, healed compression fractures), swing-away foot rests for safety during transfers, and wheel lock extensions to allow self-initiated mobility.[3,24] Make sure elderly patients fit appropriately in their chair, can reach the handrims, and can successfully disengage wheel locks to maximize independence.

- Adjustable height armrest to facilitate transfers
- Padded, wide, flat armrests[8]
- Back insert to accommodate any fixed kyphosis[24]
- Swing-away footrests for safe transfers[24]
- Pressure-relieving seat cushion[24]
- Incontinence seat covers
- Consider restraint policies on positioning devices.

Muscular Dystrophy

The muscular dystrophy patient may need a lumbar pad and adjustable full-length armrests to support a lumbar lordosis if one exists. Future plans for power mobility should be considered.

- Lumbar support if excessive lordosis exists
- Full-length armrests for support of a lordosis[23]
- Growth capability
- Adjustable height armrests for children[18]

Cerebral Palsy

Depending on the degree of involvement, the cerebral palsy patient may need trunk support to maintain symmetry, tilt or reclined positioning for poor head and trunk control, a pressure-reducing cushion, and growth capability built into the wheelchair.

- Manual or power mobility
- Growth capability[2]: adjustable height armrests for growth;[18] growth tail on seat insert
- Postural support: seat insert, back insert, lateral trunk supports
- Pressure-reducing cushion
- Incontinence seat covers if incontinent

Premature Infant with Neurological Involvement (Cerebral Palsy)

The premature infant with neurological insult may need postural inserts to prevent deformity and a stroller with growth capability for mobility.

- Stroller
- Postural inserts
- Growth capability[2]

Precautions

Determine whether the patient is subject to any activity or positioning restrictions.[23] Two examples include restriction on self-propulsion due to exertion for the severely compromised cardiac patient or avoidance of hip flexion for the recent total hip replacement patient. The former may need power mobility (a scooter) to minimize exertion whereas the latter may need thick cushions to discourage hip flexion.

Prognosis

What will the future bring? Familiarize yourself with the progression of the disease.[23,24] Will the patient make a quick full recovery or require chronic care, or is he or she in the terminal stages of a disease? Renting a standard wheelchair may be sufficient for temporary use[23] if you anticipate the patient may not survive or alternatively will make a full recovery. For example, a patient with a fractured femur who needs a wheelchair to conserve energy or for safety due to balance problems during the healing process would rent. Such is also the case for a patient in the terminal stages of cancer.

On the other hand, purchasing a wheelchair may be appropriate if the patient's condition will be long-term. A child with cerebral palsy who does not walk will probably require long-term use of a wheelchair and may need custom-fitted postural seating inserts that can be adjusted for future body growth. Issues of durability and cosmesis become more important for long-term equipment users.[23]

Finally, if the patient has a chronic progressive deteriorating disability such as multiple sclerosis or muscular dystrophy, then purchasing a wheelchair that can be modified as the patient changes may be wise. Consider adding on components and the eventual possibility of power mobility.[23]

- *Acute disability/short-term disability*—Rent
- *End stages of terminal illness*—Rent
- *Chronic disability*—Purchase
- *Progressive deterioration*—Adjustable equipment; follow up for needed modifications

Surgeries

Are there plans for a surgery? Orthopedic surgery may alter the patient's anatomy; for example, surgical repair of a congenital hip dislocation can result in improved range of motion or a change in leg length. It may be prudent to wait until after surgery to evaluate the patient for a wheelchair because body shape and seating needs may be different following the surgery.

- *Surgery anticipated*—Consider postponing evaluation until after surgery. Alternatively, reevaluate following the surgery.
- *No surgery anticipated*—Evaluate.

Physical Rehabilitation

Is the patient currently making gains in therapy? If gains are being made in rehabilitation, the patient may no longer need a special wheelchair feature or a wheelchair at all in the near future. For example, if UE function for self-propulsion improves significantly, a manual wheelchair should be considered in lieu of a power wheelchair. Or if sitting balance is improving from fair to good, lateral trunk supports may no longer be required. In each case, it may be sensible to wait until the patient's functional level plateaus before ordering the wheelchair.[25]

Medications

Does the patient take medication that can impair his or her judgment or level of consciousness?[26] Medication can affect patient performance in a wheelchair by altering level of consciousness, motor abilities, sensibilities, or endurance level. Patients who take medications that impair judgment should be cautioned against operating a power wheelchair just as individuals who take medications that induce drowsiness are cautioned against driving a car or operating machinery.

Antiepileptic Drugs

- *Phenobarbital*—Sedation
- *Dilantin*—Visual, cerebellar-vestibular effects
- *Tegretol*—Drowsiness, vertigo, ataxia, diplopia
- *Zarontin*—Drowsiness, lethargy
- *Klonopin*—Drowsiness

Spasticity and Skeletal Muscle Relaxants

- *Baclofen*—Drowsiness, muscle weakness
- *Chlorzoxazone*—Sedation
- *Diazepam (Valium)*—Drowsiness

Antipsychotic Drug

- *Thorazine*—Extrapyramidal (akinesia, muscle rigidity, tremors)

Sedative-Hypnotics

- *Barbiturates*—Drowsiness, central nervous system (CNS) depression
- *Benzodiazepines*—Drowsiness

Medications That Predispose Patients to Bleeding
Medications that thin the blood can lead to excessive bruising in extremities that bang into hard metal wheelchair components. These components should be padded.

- *Nonsteroidal anti-inflammatory drugs (NSAIDs)*
- *Heparin*
- *Coumadin*

Alcohol or Recreational Drugs May Impair Judgment

Orthotics

Are orthotics worn while in the wheelchair? Orthotics such as long leg braces and/or a body jacket will take up space in a seating system and must be accounted for when measuring the patient for a wheelchair. Body jackets will require additional seat depth. Long leg braces may require additional seat width.

- Measure for wheelchair while the patient is wearing orthotics.

Systems Review

Are there related medical problems? Reviewing each organ system in the patient's body is a good way to cover all the bases and thereby reduce the chances of missing important information related to wheelchair needs. Thoroughness usually pays off in the end. To save time, this information may be gleaned in the patient's medical chart. Alternatively, the patient or a family member can complete an intake form in the waiting area that includes information about related medical problems.

Congenital and Hereditary

Are there skeletal deformities? The size of the patient's head may be hydrocephalic or microcephalic and require different size headrests. A child with spina bifida may have a congenital scoliosis that requires pressure relief around the spine and ribs because of the associated back deformity. A child with a congenitally shortened leg length may require a seat cushion that is cut back on the involved side. A child with a congenital hip dislocation may need a seat cushion that provides sufficient pressure relief around the involved hip region if peak interface pressures are present.

- *Hip dislocation*—Seat cushion for pressure reduction around the head of the femur
- *Scoliosis*—Custom molded back insert to accommodate fixed back deformity
- *Leg length discrepancy*—Split seat insert to accommodate a shorter thigh; adjust footplate heights if needed

Hematological

Is there a bleeding disorder? Bruising can occur when a patient body part bumps into a metal component of the wheelchair. This is a particularly relevant issue in patients with low or inhibited platelet activity due to hemophilia or thrombocytopenia.[26] Hard exposed wheelchair parts such as front rigging may require padding to minimize risk of future bruising.

Is there anemia? Patients with anemia can have limited endurance. Consider energy-conserving measures such as use of lightweight frames, a well-configured wheel axle placement in a manual wheelchair, or power mobility to conserve energy.

Cardiovascular

Is there angina or shortness of breath upon exertion? Self-propulsion may not be an option if upper extremity activity precipitates symptoms such as angina and causes damage to heart muscle. Consider energy-conserving measures such as a power mobility device.

Is there lower limb edema? Edematous feet may take up space and may therefore require larger footplates. Elevating leg rests have historically been recommended for LE edema.[7] Contrary to popular belief, there is no evidence that elevating leg rests will help reduce LE edema.

Pulmonary

Is breathing labored? If yes and manual propulsion is possible, consider energy-conserving measures such as a lightweight frame. Avoid excessive thoracic pressure from wheelchair components such as chest harnesses or lateral trunk supports, which may interfere with rib and abdominal expansion during breathing.

Is there a tracheostomy tube? Maintain the opening of the tracheostomy unobstructed. Wheelchair components such as chest harnesses and straps should not obstruct this opening. In addition, avoid positioning the patient's neck in excessive flexion, which may cause the chin to cover the tracheostomy opening.

Is oxygen or a ventilator in use? Consider attachment/storage sites for this type of equipment onto the wheelchair.[21]

Gastrointestinal

Is there bowel incontinence? Consider fecal-resistant upholstery such as vinyl on the seat. Open cell seat cushions (such as T foam) allow penetration of liquids and should be covered with a protective washable cover. Guard against the negative presence of moisture (i.e., feces) on pressure ulcers. Be aware of colostomy bag location if present.

Is there gastroesophageal (GE) reflux?[14] If GE reflux is present, one goal for the patient may be an upright seated position.

Is there a gastrostomy tube? Avoid pressure from seat belts and straps that may stretch or occlude the gastrostomy tube as it exits the patient's abdomen. Consider ordering and attaching a feeding pole to the wheelchair for patients who are continuously fed by a feeding tube.

Is there weight gain? Patients may suffer from ascites, bloating, obesity, or organ enlargement. If the patient occupies a lot of space in a seat or is very heavy, consider width, depth, and strength requirements of the wheelchair. Make sure the manufacturer of the wheelchair frame warrantees the chair to withstand loads up to the client's body weight. Consider reclining the back insert a little to improve comfort and reduce pressure between the patient's thighs and abdomen if compression is present.

Is there weight loss? Soft tissue helps to pad our bones. If the patient loses weight, adipose tissue will be reduced and bony areas under pressure such as the ischia may be more susceptible to pressure ulcer development. Frail individuals have a higher risk for pressure ulcers.[15] Consider padding the metal portion of the seat belt buckle to avoid concentrated forces over bony pelvic areas such as the anterior superior iliac spines. Sufficiently cushion the seat under the bony ischia and greater trochanters.

Are there weight fluctuations over time? If weight fluctuates, be cautious about recommending custom fitted components like molded back inserts, which cannot be altered later. Custom fitted components may fit well today but poorly next month following a precipitous weight gain or loss. In these cases, consider wheelchair components that are adjustable; for example, lateral trunk supports can be designed with knobs that can be adjusted in or out in width to accommodate changing trunk girth.

Urologic

Is there urinary incontinence? Consider urine-resistant upholstery such as vinyl over the seat cushion. Consider closed cell foams that don't allow liquids to penetrate.

Is there frequent urination? Consider wheelchair components such as front rigging, armrests, and wheel locks that are easy to manage for quick transfers to a toilet.

Are there external urinary bags, tubes, or catheters? Avoid pressure from seat belts and straps at these sites because pressure can occlude tube drainage.

Gynecological

Is the patient pregnant? Consider accommodating short-term growth changes in the wheelchair for the patient. For example, recline the back a little to reduce pressure between thighs and abdomen if the patient does not tolerate an upright position. Consider extra long seat belts as the pregnancy progresses. Order adjustable height armrests to facilitate patient transfers into and out of the wheelchair.

Nutritional and Metabolic

Is osteoporosis/osteopenia present? Avoid concentrated forces over bones that may lead to fractures. Ankle straps that secure a foot on a footrest may result in excessive forces around the tibia if the patient pushes out against the strap. Consider padding a footbox to protect the feet from kicking activity rather than using ankle straps if osteoporosis is present. Alternatively, distribute force over a larger surface area so pressure is reduced in bony areas at risk of fracturing. During two-person maximal assisted transfers, consider having the patient wear a temporary/transfer splint on body parts at risk of fracturing in order to reduce stress from the weight of the limb on the bones. These splints can be removed following the transfer.

Endocrine

Is there diabetes?[14] Protect the patient from sustaining sores and cuts from wheelchair components because wounds may heal poorly. Diabetes is also a risk factor for pressure ulceration.

Are there associated growth disturbances? Patients with short UEs may require adjustable rear wheel axles, a narrower frame, cambered wheels, or larger wheels in order to facilitate reach of the wheels for self-propulsion. On the other hand, patients with short LEs may require a frame that is low to the floor to facilitate transfers into the wheelchair.

Musculoskeletal/Connective Tissue

Are there contractures? Limited joint mobility in the hips and knees may prevent a patient from fitting into a standard wheelchair. If the patient has less than 90 degrees of hip flexion, the back of the frame may have to be reclined. If the patient has knee flexion contractures, the feet may need to be supported under the seat of the wheelchair. If the patient has an equinus deformity at the ankles, angle-adjustable footrests may be necessary to support the feet.

Is there muscle, joint, or bone pain? If LE pain significantly limits walking, a wheelchair may be indicated for long distance transportation. If UE pain limits manual wheelchair propulsion, a lighter frame, better chair configuration, or power mobility may be required.

Has the patient been inactive or on bedrest? Bedrest weakens most body systems, deconditions the cardiovascular system, and can lead to disuse atrophy in skeletal muscle. Muscle strength, aerobic endurance, and bone strength may be affected, resulting in deteriorated patient performance during transfers, walking, and wheelchair activities. If a new wheelchair is being considered, and you believe the patient's abilities will markedly improve, consider conducting the wheelchair evaluation after the patient is reconditioned/recovers from the effects of bedrest.

PATIENT HISTORY

Adjusting to an upright position may need to be accomplished gradually using a recliner, backward tilt-in-space wheelchair, or tilt table.

Neurologic

How alert is the patient? A diminished level of consciousness may not be compatible with safe, independent skills such as power mobility.

Are there seizures? If the patient has a seizure, he or she may lose control of motor abilities temporarily. Make sure the patient is adequately protected from injuries during uncontrolled movements. Power mobility may not be a safe option for patients who have petit mal or grand mal seizures.

Is there sensory loss? Consider using pressure-reducing cushion materials that help distribute pressure in areas that are insensate and have the potential for skin breakdown. Teach pressure relief maneuvers.

Is there uncontrolled movement? Anticipate sites of potential injuries as a result of uncontrolled movements (e.g., Huntington's chorea). Pad wheelchair parts as needed.

Is there the potential for nonverbal communication? Consider consulting with a communication specialist (speech and language pathologist) for appropriate technology that can be used while the patient is in the wheelchair.[27]

Does the patient have difficulty handling saliva? Consider easy to clean fabrics for the seating system. Consider consulting with a speech and language pathologist to improve the patient's ability to handle saliva.

Is there a temperature regulation problem? If the patient experiences fluctuations in body temperature, make sure there is sufficient space in the seating system for periodic use or removal of additional clothing, blankets, or thermal equipment. Note that custom molded seating inserts closely fit around the patient's trunk and may not offer sufficient space for additional clothing.

Psychiatric/Psychological

Is the patient a danger to him/herself or others? Consider nonremovable components such as armrests, brake extensions, and front rigging so they cannot be used as weapons.

Is there self-abuse? Protect the patient from harm by padding or removing hard or sharp components. For example, if the patient bangs his or her head into the lap board, the board should be either padded or removed.

Are there behavior problems? If the patient can walk, but refuses, a wheelchair or stroller (depending on age) may be useful temporarily to enable the patient to attend clinics. I once had a parent complain of how her child (with walking difficulties) would refuse to ambulate any further to an appointment and intentionally drop to the ground. The child presented with thick knee calluses bilaterally.

Are there specific restraint policies where the patient resides? In nursing homes, equipment like seat belts and lap boards may not be permitted on a patient's wheelchair if the equipment is viewed as a restraint. Check whether restraint policies prohibit the use of positioning equipment.

Dermatological

Is there contact dermatitis? Certain materials like industrial chemicals and metals may cause a skin reaction or rash in the patient when they contact the skin. Commonly affected skin areas include the face, neck, hands, legs, and feet. Avoid materials (e.g., metals, fabrics, latex) that the patient is hypersensitive to, or cover these parts during wheelchair construction.[28]

Social History

Lifestyle

Where Will the Patient Be Living?

The patient's residence must be wheelchair accessible. Three common access problems include the entry into the home, up the stairs, and in the bathrooms.[29] A patient who lives in a house or an apartment may need ramps, wider doors, and other home renovations. A patient who lives in a residential facility may already have full access to all areas in the building. Hallways need to be wide enough to allow a wheelchair to turn around a corner. Bathroom doorways need to be wide enough to clear a rolling commode chair. Tables need to be high enough to allow the patient's knees to fit under the table.

- *Facilities*—May be wheelchair accessible
- *Private houses and apartments*—May have architectural barriers and require planning for narrower, lighter, or folding wheelchairs and/or home renovation

Who Will Be Caring for the Patient?

As a general rule, the more people involved in the patient's care, the more difficult it will be to take care of patient property like a wheelchair. If many people take care of the patient (three nursing shifts, school, bus driver), there is a good chance wheelchair parts will get lost. Consider having the patient's name written on all removable parts. Try to reduce the number of components that can be removed from the wheelchair to minimize loss. Teach all persons involved in the patient's care how to handle the wheelchair properly.

- *Many people*—Greater chance of lost property: place name labels on equipment
- *Few people*—More consistent care of property
- *Patient lives alone*—Order low-maintenance equipment[24]

How Many Hours Does the Patient Spend in a Wheelchair

Break down the patient's day into thirds and determine how the patient's morning, afternoon, and evening are spent. How many rest periods does the patient need out of the wheelchair? Does the patient stay in bed most of the time or remain in the wheelchair all day? If the patient spends a minimal amount of time in a wheelchair, customized postural supports may not be crucial. On the other hand, if the patient spends many hours in a wheelchair, a pressure-reducing cushion and postural supports become increasingly more important for comfort, support (to prevent deformity), and pressure reduction (to prevent pressure ulcers).

- *Minimal time in wheelchair*—Custom postural support may not be critical
- *Many hours in wheelchair*—Pressure-reducing cushion and postural support become increasingly more important

What Duties Are Required of the Patient?

This question immediately places the patient's problems into a meaningful context. For example, does the patient need a standing frame to perform duties at work, a power wheelchair or ultralight frame to travel across town, or a power tilt-in-space mechanism to provide a rest period so that long hours at a job or in school can be tolerated?

Indoor/Outdoor Environments

Will the Patient Spend Most of the Time Indoors or Outdoors?

A patient who mostly remains indoors will deal with a less physically and perceptually demanding environment. On the other hand, a patient who ventures outdoors must deal with a more challenging and less predictable environment including oncoming cars, uneven terrain, and changing weather conditions.[30]

Indoors

Patients may not require a heavy-duty wheelchair if it will solely be used indoors and the patient is not particularly rough on the frame. Determine if the patient's home is wheelchair accessible (Figure 2-1). Have the patient or family draw a layout of the home if important room, corridor, or furniture dimensions are not clear.

Door Openings

Measure the maximum width of door openings to ensure that the wheelchair, and lap board if used, can fit through doorways. The recommended doorway clearance

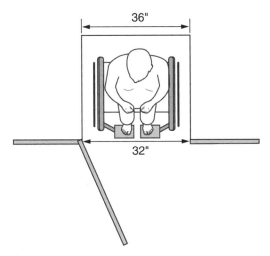

FIGURE 2-1 Wheelchair accessibility. A 32-inch doorway and 36-inch corridor clearance is sufficient for most wheelchairs. Determine maximal doorway clearance with the door open by measuring from the door jamb on one side (vertical side piece of the opening) to the inside corner of the door.

needed for a standard wheelchair is 32 inches.[31] This amount of clearance should be sufficient for a 26-inch-wide standard adult wheelchair. Bathroom doorways are typically too narrow for a wheelchair. Bariatric patients may need a wider clearance.

- Recommended door opening clearance—32 inches[31,32]
- Standard wheelchair width—26 inches[31]

Corridors
Measure corridor width to determine if a wheelchair has sufficient width for passage.

- Minimal passage width for one wheelchair—36 inches (32 inches to pass a short distance)[31]
- Minimal passage width for two wheelchairs—60 inches[31]
- Minimal width for one ambulator to pass one wheelchair—48 inches[31]

Clearance on Turns
Make sure the wheelchair will have enough room to make a turn (180-degree angle) in a narrow hallway. Turning requires an area with a 60-inch diameter.[31] The longer a wheelchair frame is, the more difficult it will be to negotiate turns in

a narrow hallway. Turns will be more difficult if elevated leg rests are used because they make the wheelchair longer.

- Turning space required for a standard wheelchair—60-inch diameter[31]

Work Surfaces
Measure work surface height for clearance of knees under the work surface. Work surfaces need to be at least 27 inches off the floor to clear the knee of an individual in a standard adult wheelchair. More knee clearance may be needed if thicker seat cushions are used or the seat level is raised.

- Height of tables—range from 28 to 34 inches from floor[31] (for standard wheelchair)
- Knee clearance—at least 27 (ht) × 30 (w) × 19 inches (d).[31]

Bed Height
Determine the difference between wheelchair seat height and bed height during transfers.[23] The seat level on a standard adult wheelchair is 19 inches.[31] A seat cushion, however, may raise the seat height. A hospital bed with adjustable height features may be able to level the bed mattress to the same height of the seat cushion to facilitate sliding board transfers. Elevating wheelchairs can facilitate sliding board transfers to different bed heights.

Floor Surface
If floors are carpeted, consider pneumatic tires and casters to reduce rolling resistance of the wheelchair.[24] For hard indoor surfaces, solid tires are adequate.

Size of Rooms
Bedrooms should have adequate space to maneuver a wheelchair around in preparation of transfers. The minimal space required for one stationary wheelchair and user is 30 × 48 inches.[31]

Elevator or Stairs
Minimal elevator dimensions to fit a standard wheelchair are 51 × 36 inches.[31] If the elevator is frequently out of order and the family lives on a high floor in an apartment building, the family may need to carry the wheelchair up several flights of stairs. Consider a lighter weight wheelchair with detachable components or a stroller for these patients. Rehabilitation Engineering and Assistive Technology Society of America (RESNA) wheelchair standards offer guidelines for reporting the weight of frames and each component.

Small Living Spaces
For studio living, order a wheelchair that folds in order to take up less space. The width of a folded standard adult wheelchair is 11 inches.[32] Consider ordering an indoor wheelchair with large wheels in the front for better maneuverability in a small living space.

Architectural Barriers in the Home

Consider the following options if a wheelchair is required but the home is inaccessible:

- Order the narrowest frame width possible to clear doorway openings.
- Order a lightweight frame (or appropriate size stroller with postural insert/ transport chair if patient does not self-propel) to carry on stairs.
- Order detachable components to make the wheelchair lighter while carrying on stairs.
- Remove handrims if patient does not self-propel to clear doorway openings.
- Order wraparound or fixed (nonremovable) armrests to minimize width.
- Do not camber the rear wheels to minimize width.
- Order a narrowing device to temporarily narrow frame width to clear doorways.
- Order a folding frame to clear doorway openings with the patient out of the wheelchair.
- Renovate the home or find accessible housing.
- Refer the patient to social worker/case worker for housing assistance.

Outdoors

Stronger wheelchair construction is generally recommended for rugged outdoor use. Consider having the patient or family draw a map of the neighborhood including important places and distances (city blocks). The following areas may be included:

- *Destinations*—Important destinations for the patient (bus stop, work, bank, grocery store, restaurants, clinic, school, park)
- *Distances*—How far to travel to important destinations
- *Time*—How much time it takes to get to a destination
- *Type of terrain*—The type of wheelchair construction (standard, lightweight, heavy duty) and tires will be determined in part by where the wheelchair will be used.
  - *Bumpy terrain*[24] *(grass, gravel)*—Consider pneumatic or wide tires for greater shock absorption; heavy-duty or strong frame construction and large casters to negotiate over cracks.
  - *Broken glass*—Consider no air (no flat) tires for maintenance-free care.
  - *Hilly terrain*—Consider a lightweight manual frame; make sure power wheelchairs can negotiate steep hills. Grade aid wheel locks may assist manual negotiations up hills.
  - *Inclines*—To prevent backward tipping on inclines, consider anti-tippers, a long anterior/posterior frame base of support, an amputee frame, or a posterior rear wheel axial position.[24] RENSA wheelchair standards offer stability tests that indicate how stable a chair is while on an inclined surface.[33]
  - *Ramps*—The minimal width for standard wheelchair clearance on ramps is 36 inches.[31]

- *How will the patient be transported?*—If the patient uses the bus, make sure the wheelchair is narrow enough to get on the ramp and low enough for the patient and wheelchair to clear the top of the bus or van door. Also make sure the wheelchair is capable of being secured (tied-down) to the floor of the vehicle properly for safety. Consider the use of a headrest (removable) to reduce risk of whiplash in a wheelchair during bus travel. Order transit options on a new wheelchair that have been crash tested and are WC-19 compliant.[34]

If the patient travels by car or taxi, consider wheelchair weight, make sure the wheelchair folds easily, and think about ordering removable rear wheels (quick release wheels) to facilitate storage during transportation.

Funding Source

Explore all potential funding sources with a case worker because wheelchair recommendations may ultimately be constrained by available funds.[23]

Exercises

1. Discuss prescription considerations based on patient age, gender, body weight, and height.
2. What kind of wheelchair prescription might a clinician first consider for the following diagnoses?
   a. High tetraplegia
   b. Cerebral vascular accident
   c. Amputation
   d. Paraplegia
   e. Self-abuse
3. What medications might interfere with a patient's safe operation of power mobility?
4. Conduct a systems review and consider how each system may impact your decision to prescribe a wheelchair.
5. How would a patient with an acute, chronic, or progressive condition affect your decision to prescribe a wheelchair?

References

1. McDonald R, Surtees R, Wirz S. A comparison between parents' and therapists' views of their child's individual seating systems. *Int J Rehabil Res.* 2003;26:235–243.
2. Freney D. Pediatric seating. *Home Health Care Dealer/Supplier.* 1995;Sept/Oct:103–105.
3. Dworak P, Folland R, Kirkner A. Age of matter. *Rehabil Manage.* 2004;December:26–29.
4. Fay BT, Thorman TA, Cooper R. The yin and yang of wheelchair use: addressing gender-based differences in manual wheelchair users. Available at: http://www.rehabpub .com/ltrehab/32001/2.asp. Accessed October 29, 2008.
5. Boninger ML, Dicianno BE, Cooper RA, Towers JD, Koontz AM, Souza AL. Shoulder magnetic resonance imaging abnormalities, wheelchair propulsion, and gender. *Arch Phys Med Rehabil.* 2003;84(11):1615–1620. Erratum in: *Arch Phys Med Rehabil.* 2004;85(1):172.
6. Reid D, Angus J, McKeever P, Miller K-L. Home is where their wheels are: experiences of women wheelchair users. *Am J Occup Ther.* 2003;57(2):186–195.
7. Wilson AB, McFarland SR. Types of wheelchairs. *J Rehabil Res Dev.* 1990;2(Supp):104–116.
8. Redford JB. Seating and wheeled mobility in the disabled elderly population. *Arch Phys Med Rehabil.* 1993;74:877–885.
9. Collinger JL, Boninger ML, Koontz AM, et al. Shoulder biomechanics during the push phase of wheelchair propulsion: a multisite study of persons with paraplegia. *Arch Phys Med Rehabil.* 2008;89(4):667–676.
10. Mercer JL, Boninger M, Koontz A, Ren D, Dyson-Hudson T, Cooper R. Shoulder joint kinetics and pathology in manual wheelchair users. *Clin Biomech.* 2006;21(8):781–789.
11. Boninger ML, Cooper RA, Baldwin MA, Shimada SD, Koontz A. Wheelchair pushrim kinetics: body weight and median nerve function. *Arch Phys Med Rehabil.* 1999;80(8):910–915.

PATIENT HISTORY

12. Diconsiglio J. Hospitals equip to meet the bariatric challenge. *Materials Manage Health Care.* 2006;April:36–39.

13. U.S. Access Board. Americans with Disabilities Act (ADA) and Architectural Barriers Act accessibility guidelines. July 23, 2004. Available at: http://www.access-board.gov/ada-aba/final.pdf. Accessed October 29, 2008.

14. Currie DM, Hardwick K, Marburger RA, Britell CW. Wheelchair prescription and adaptive seating. In Delisa JL, Gans BM, eds. *Rehabilitation Medicine: Principles and Practice,* 2nd ed. Philadelphia: JB Lippincott; 1993:563–585.

15. Garber SL, Krouskop TA. Body build and its relationship to pressure distribution in the seated wheelchair patient. *Arch Phys Med Rehabil.* 1982;63:17–20.

16. Webster JS, Rapport LJ, Godlewski MC, Abadee PS. Effect of attentional bias to right space on wheelchair mobility. *J Clin Exp Neuropsychol.* 1994;16(1):129–137.

17. Brattström M, Brattström H, Eklöf M, Fredström J. The rheumatoid patient in need of a wheelchair. *Scand J Rehabil Med.* 1981;13:39–43.

18. Bergen AF, Presperin J, Tallman T. *Positioning for Function: Wheelchairs and Other Assistive Technologies.* Valhalla, NY: Valhalla Rehabilitation; 1990:13–82.

19. Cooper RA, Fitzgerald SG, Boninger ML, et al. Evaluation of a pushrim-activated, power-assisted wheelchair. *Arch Phys Med Rehabil.* 2001;82:702–708.

20. Kohlmeyer KM, Yarkony GM. Functional outcomes after spinal cord injury rehabilitation. In Yarkony GM, ed. *Spinal Cord Injury: Medical Management and Rehabilitation.* Gaithersburg, MD: Aspen; 1994:9–14.

21. Warren CG. Technical considerations: power mobility and its implications. *J Rehabil Res Dev.* 1990;2(Supp):74-85.

22. Ragnarsson KT. Clinical perspectives on wheelchair selection: prescription considerations and a comparison of conventional and light weight wheelchairs. *J Rehabil Res Dev.* 1990;2(Supp):8–16.

23. Mattingly D. Wheelchair selection. *Orthop Nurs.* 1993;12:11–17.

24. Behrman AL. Clinical perspectives on wheelchair selection: factors in functional assessment. *J Rehabil Res Dev.* 1990;2(Supp):17–27.

25. Batavia M, Gianutsos JG, Kambouris M. An augmented auditory feedback device. *Arch Phys Med Rehab.* 1997;78(12):1389–1392.

26. Eddy L. *Physical Therapy Pharmacology.* St Louis, MO: Mosby Year Book; 1992:73–79, 107–125.

27. Taylor SJ. Evaluating the client with physical disabilities for wheelchair sitting. *Am J Occup Ther.* 1987;41:711–716.

28. Marino MA, Vivio SDR. Care of children with physical and emotional problems. In Christensen B, Kockrow E, eds. *Foundations of Nursing.* St Louis, MO: Mosby; 1995:1369–1446.

29. Pynoos J, Overton J. A changing environment. *Rehabil Manage.* 2003;16(2):38–42.

30. Poulton EC. On prediction in skilled movements. *Psychol Bull.* 1957;54:467–478.

31. American National Standards Institute. *American National Standard for Buildings and Facilities: Providing Accessibility and Usability for Physically Handicapped People. Accessible Elements and Spaces (A117.1).* New York: American National Standards Institute; 1986:16–73.

32. Olson SC, Meredith DK. *Wheelchair Interiors.* Chicago: National Easter Seal Society; 1973:3–16.

33. The ANSI/RESNA wheelchair standards: sample evaluation and guide to interpreting test data for prescribing power wheelchairs. *Health Devices.* 1993;22(10):432–484.

34. Zimmerman JM. Get on the bus. *Rehabil Manage.* 2003;16(7):48–51, 74.

CHAPTER 3

Clinical Examination

The clinical exam identifies physical impairments that can affect wheelchair abilities. For example, a hip joint extension contracture will affect a patient's ability to sit. Upper extremity (UE) pain may affect the patient's ability to propel a wheelchair.

The assessment involves a sitting exam and a mat exam. Why two exams? By doing both you get a more complete picture of how the patient behaves under varied gravitational conditions. Although sitting simulates real world conditions under gravity, recumbency will *reveal* truncal dimensions, joint mobility, reflex activity, and postural alignment possibilities under a less strenuous, gravity-eliminated situation. You may need a second clinician to assist during portions of the sitting and mat examinations.

Components of the clinical exam include anthropometrics, postural alignment, active movements, sitting balance, muscle tone/reflexes, endurance, speed, strength, perception, cognitive status, passive range of motion, skin status, and sensation. Although anthropometrics, postural alignment, sensation, and muscle tone/reflexes should be evaluated in both positions, skin inspection and range of motion are ideally performed on the mat.

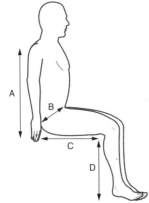

Anthropometric Measurements

Measure the patient's body dimensions in supine and sitting with a tape measure to determine the proper size wheelchair (Figure 3-1).*

Position the patient supine with the hips and knees in 90 degrees of flexion,[1] or sitting on a firm surface with feet supported on a flat surface (e.g., floor) and sufficient guarding for

FIGURE 3-1 To determine wheelchair size, measure back height (**A**), seat width (**B**), seat depth (**C**), and leg length (**D**) from knee to heel on the patient.

---

* It may be wise to check available ROM in the patient prior to measuring body dimensions in sitting.

safety. (Ask for help to support the patient if necessary.) Note that measurements may be different between sitting and supine (e.g., shorter back height in sitting) because of the gravitational effects on the trunk. Measure the patient twice to ensure reliable records. Also, measure the patient wearing any orthotics and prosthetics in use. Remember to account for seat cushion height, which may add two or more inches to the back height depending on cushion thickness, although some settling (immersion) will occur over time. Also account for postural support pieces such as hip guides and lateral trunk supports that can add width to the client in the wheelchair (usually 1 inch per side).

Wheelchair Frame Dimensions*

Seat height is the measurement from floor to seat (i.e., from the bottom of the heel to the posterior thigh)[2,3] plus two additional inches to account for footplate height from the floor.

Seat width is the measurement from hip to hip plus two additional inches.[2,3] Whenever possible, measure for the narrowest wheelchair size because patients will be able to access the rear wheels better and clear through doorways and ramps more easily. If the patient does not require postural supports to address deformity[4] and a close fit is desired,[1] seat width measurement may be the distance between the patient's greater trochanters (i.e., distance between seat rails). Orthotics, hip guides, thicker winter clothing, and anticipated weight gains, however, may require additional seat width.[1] Regardless of the patient's situation, hips should not be laterally compressed by the sides of the wheelchair.[4]

Seat depth is the measurement from the front of the seat (back of knee) to the back of the pelvis (with the pelvis touching the back of the chair). Subtract up to 2 inches from the measurement to provide clearance between the front edge of the seat and the back of the knee.[2,3] Measure each leg individually if a femoral leg length discrepancy exists. The front edge of the seat should generally be *no more than 2 inches* from the popliteal crease after the patient is properly positioned.[4]

Back height is the measurement from the seat to the level on the patient's back that will offer sufficient back support[2,3] (typically to the inferior angle of the scapula; lower if trunk control is good, higher if additional spinal support is required).[4]

Leg length is the measurement from the seat surface to the footplate.[2,3] If a leg length discrepancy exists between tibias, measure each leg individually so that each foot can be supported at different levels.

Arm height, which determines armrest height, is measured from the seat to the elbow (with the scapula relaxed, arm vertical, elbow flexed to 90 degrees, and forearm pronated). Then add 1 inch to the measurement so the upper limb is adequately supported.[2,3] Arm height is important for push off during transfers, pressure relief maneuvers, and postural support for the trunk. Account for seat cushion thickness when measuring armrest height because the cushion adds height to the seat.[3]

Additional measurements may be useful if you are measuring for other components such as placement of lateral trunk supports (chest width), harness size (i.e.,

---

* Some variation in how different manufacturers determine frame size.

trunk width and length), head supports (i.e., head width and length), or footplate size (i.e., foot length).

Postural Alignment

Ideal posture can be viewed from an evolutionary, structural, or functional perspective. From an evolutionary viewpoint, ideal posture may be the position from which the individual can respond equally well from all directions and with the least amount of energy.[5] For example, consider sitting in a chair with the intention of standing up in order to avoid danger. You will be in a better sitting posture to quickly move in any direction and with less preparation if your feet are first both planted on the floor instead of resting under the chair.

Ideal posture can also be viewed structurally as that which is symmetric. When symmetry is possible, our joints are not in extreme positions, our muscles are not working excessively to keep us upright, and we can perform movements to a similar extent on either side of the body. Some might even argue that symmetry has an esthetic appeal. Symmetry, however, does not always equate with function, so the impact of positioning should always be checked against patient outcomes (i.e., skills, abilities). Ultimately, our goal is to have patients *function maximally* in a wheelchair if they use one.

A trade-off between ideal positioning and function is illustrated in Sprigle et al.'s study that found reaching was better when spinal cord injured (SCI) wheelchair users with tetra- and paraplegia (*n* = 20) were positioned in a posterior pelvic tilt.[6] Subjects were 18 to 64 years old, had American Spinal Injury Association (ASIA) scores from 65 to 247, and were tested under different pelvic positions, cushion types, and backrest heights. Reach ability (i.e., bilateral, unilateral, horizontal sweeping across) was predicted by posture but not equipment. A more stable posterior tilt posture (an average of 16.6 degrees in this sample) may have provided a foundation for which upper trunk and UEs could function in this population. (On the flip side, posterior pelvic positioning may also have a deleterious impact on seating pressures and pressure ulcer formation.) In any case, we don't normally view a posteriorly tilted pelvis as structurally ideal, although in this case it is functional.

The importance of assessing the unique postural needs of each patient is highlighted by Bolin et al. who argued for individualized rather than "standard solutions" to sitting problems in four C5–6 SCI cases.[7] Each case required a unique postural intervention.

Assessing Postural Alignment

Step 1. Determine if the patient's pelvis is positioned to the rear of the seat. Start with the pelvis—the foundation for all sitting. Ask the patient or assist the patient to sit toward the rear of the seat so the posterior pelvic area is contacting the back of the wheelchair. You can visually confirm that the patient's posterior pelvic area is touching the back of the wheelchair by having the patient lean their trunk slightly forward so the posterior pelvis can be inspected.

Step 2. Observe how the patient sits. Check if the patient naturally assumes a balanced or symmetrical sitting posture with eyes horizontal, nose vertical, shoulders level, and pelvis level, or alternatively sits out of midline.

Step 3. Ask the patient to assume a symmetrical sitting posture. Once the patient's pelvis is to the rear of the seat, ask the patient to voluntarily sit symmetrically if he or she did not do so spontaneously.

Step 4. If the patient cannot actively sit symmetrically, can correction be attained with gentle force using external supports?[8] If the patient is flexible (i.e., easily bends without discomfort) in the neck, trunk, and pelvis, then symmetrical sitting may be possible using postural supports. Equipment should be used judiciously, however, because some patients may learn to rely on postural supports rather than on themselves to balance and sit upright. Care must also be taken not to compress pressure-sensitive structures in the axilla (brachial plexus, vessels).

A three-point force system applied with lateral thoracic supports has been used for a flexible neuromuscular scoliosis. Holmes et al. compared the immediate effects of two thoracic trunk support configurations: One with both thoracic supports positioned near the axilla and another using a three-point force configuration with one thoracic pad on the convex apex of the scoliosis and the other near the axilla on the concave side.[9] The subjects were 16 nonambulatory children* with spastic quadriplegia, cerebral palsy, and a neuromuscular scoliosis. Compared to a no thoracic support condition there was an 18.6% mean curve correction (i.e., spinous process angle) using pad supports under the axilla and a 34% mean correction using the three-point force configuration. Long-term effects and positional tolerance were not assessed in their study.

Step 5. If the patient cannot achieve symmetrical sitting with gentle force, decide on the optimal position for patient function and accommodate support around this fixed position.[10,11] If fixed deformities and asymmetries are present, such as an inflexible scoliosis or a dislocated hip, determine which body part will be oriented toward the patient's environment and position accordingly. Should the patient's head, shoulders, pelvis, knees, or feet face front? If rotational deformities are present, it will not be possible to have all body parts oriented in a forward-facing direction.

One approach is to orient the patient's head toward the midline and balance the head and trunk over the pelvis. Get the head and shoulders level and facing front if possible with the eyes horizontal and the nose is vertical[10] (Figure 3-2). The sense organs for vision, hearing, taste, and smell are located in the head and should be oriented toward the patient's environment so that the patient can optimally interact. Remaining body parts, such as the pelvis, hips, knees, and feet, should then be supported in whatever posture they are fixed in. In any case, avoid excessive weight bearing over one ischium when attempting to balance the patient's head and shoulders over an inflexible spine.

---

* Ages 6.5–20.8 years; 9 boys, 7 girls; all were also provided with lateral pelvic support pads.

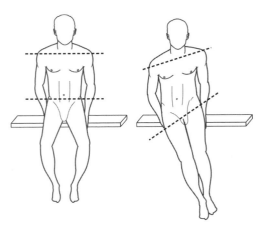

FIGURE 3-2
(A) Symmetrical sitting with nose vertical, eyes horizontal, and shoulders and iliac crest level.
(B) In patients with fixed asymmetrical deformity, the head is balanced over the support base with eyes horizontal and nose vertical.

Patients with significant scoliosis may have to position their lower limbs in a windswept position (both knees deviated off to the same side) so their head and eyes are allowed to face front (Figure 3-3). *It is important* that the patient and family are prepared for this approach because existing rotational deformities may appear more conspicuous.

Active Movement

Is Any Movement Possible?

If the patient is completely paralyzed, there is a great risk for skin breakdown because weight shifting, which relieves pressure, will not be possible. Teach weight-shifting activities to patients who can move; have caregivers change the patient's position periodically for patients who cannot. Consider a pressure-reducing seat cushion. Reclining and tilt-in-space wheelchair frames can also help to shift the patient's weight-bearing area in the seat.[12]

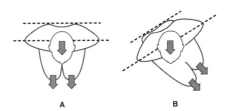

FIGURE 3-3 (A) Patient is symmetrical with head, shoulders, and hips facing front. **(B)** Patient exhibits a fixed windswept deformity and must have hips positioned out of midline so the head can remain facing front.

If Movement Is Not Possible

- Attendant-assisted pressure relief[13]
- Independent weight shifts using a power tilt or recline on frame[14]

If Movement Is Possible

- Teach independent pressure relief[13,15]

If the Patient Is Active, Are Movements Rich and Varied?

One of the hallmarks of physical disability, especially with brain damage, is a reduction in the richness or variety of voluntary movements that able-body individuals normally possess. The stereotypic lower extremity scissoring activity in cerebral palsy or the persistently flexed posture in Parkinson's disease are quintessential examples of the poverty of movement associated with patients who have central nervous system dysfunction. Although movement variety may be small, some voluntary movements can be put to good use. Determine what movements are possible for the patient and then attempt to assist the patient in using these movements to capitalize on function.

Are Movements Functional and Reliable?

Determine what useful movements are consistently within the patient's repertoire and could be put to good use if matched with the appropriate equipment. For example, could the patient's hands or feet be used to propel the wheelchair if the wheel was closer to the hand or the seat lower to the floor? Could the patient open and fasten the seat belt if an airplane-type belt was provided? Could a patient with only head movement adopt a more independent lifestyle if a strategically placed switch was placed on a headrest to permit power wheelchair operation? Note that patients with only $3/16$ of an inch of available movement may be able to operate a control switch on a power wheelchair.[14]

Maximize the function potential of reliable movements using assistive technologies and switches.[14] Consult with occupational therapy (OT) and assistive technology experts.

Are One or Two Body Movements Available for Operating the Controls of a Power Wheelchair?[14]

- Tongue control
- Puff/sip control
- Chin control
- Headrest control
- Manual joystick
- Arm/elbow control
- Shoulder position
- Lip control

- Knee control
- Foot control

Can Movements Result in Injury?

Not all movements are functional. The problem is when movement-related injuries occur while in a wheelchair. Injuries are common in patients with Huntington's disease, for example, because of their incessant choreic movements.

Before dispensing the wheelchair, determine if any body segment is at risk for harm. Systematically survey the patient's movement repertoire from head to toe to determine if any of these moving body segments can potentially result in wheelchair-related injuries or fatalities. Pad components or block movement that can lead to injury, and inspect the patient's environment for hazardous conditions (e.g., stairs).

Survey body areas at risk of injury from head to toe:

- *The head* can get caught around a headrest if the patient tends to list his or her trunk to the side of the headrest.
- *The neck* can get hung up in the chest harness if the patient has poor sitting control and slides forward in the wheelchair.
- *The upper limbs* could fall behind a lap board or the fingers could get caught in the wheelchair spokes.
- *The trunk* can get bruised from leaning over the armrest if the patient has poor trunk control.
- *The feet* can fall off the footplate and drag on the ground.
- *The wheelchair may tip* in any direction.
- *Inspect the environment* for high-risk areas.

Environmental Factors Associated with Wheelchair-Related Fatalities[16]

- Stairs—most common
- Bathroom
- Ramps
- Water
- Cars
- Curb
- Elevator, train tracks, garage door

Injuries Associated with Wheelchair-Related Fatalities[16]

- Skeletal—most common, especially femoral fractures
- Respiratory
- Nervous
- Cardiovascular
- Integumentary
- Gastrointestinal; genitourinary

Does the Patient Get Stuck in One Position or Can the Patient Reverse Direction Without Assistance?

Can the patient safely move into and out of a position without help? It may be okay for patients to temporarily hook their head around the side of a headrest and then return to their original position, but not acceptable if they are stuck in that posture for an hour. At issue is whether the patient becomes trapped in a dangerous position. If the patient cannot reverse the direction of a movement, then consider blocking (stopping) that movement with adaptive equipment such as lateral trunk supports until the patient can achieve better control.

Are UE Degenerative Changes Associated with Wheelchair Use?

Long-term use of a wheelchair could lead to wear and tear (repetitive) upper extremity injuries such as osteoarthritis, rotator cuff injuries, bursitis, and tenosynovitis.[17]

Sitting Balance (Righting and Equilibrium)

Can the Patient Sit Without External Support?

Determine if the patient sits safely under static and dynamic conditions because both may be encountered during a patient's day. Can the patient respond quickly to the perturbation or is the response too slow or delayed to be of safe functional value? Perturbations can also occur during abrupt power mobility accelerations or while traveling over rough terrain and curbs. If responses to perturbations are inadequate or too challenging, postural supports such as a chest harness or lateral trunk supports may be necessary for safety. Also, limits to speed using power mobility may be required.

Static Sitting Balance

Static sitting balance is determined by first having the patient short sit with feet supported on the floor while the patient is adequately guarded by someone. Then explain the procedure to the patient and gently push the patient in anterior, posterior, and lateral directions while you observe how the patient recovers from the perturbation. Can the patient maintain his or her eyes and shoulders horizontal during the perturbation or does the patient's head and trunk list uncontrollable to the side? Can the patient recover from the perturbation without the assistance of the clinician?

Alternatively, have the patient sit on a base that tilts and perturb the base of support to observe how the patient recovers when suddenly moved. (This test may simulate balance demands in a moving vehicle like a bus.) Even better, observe trunk control/balance under real-life conditions (e.g., vehicle transportation), provided sufficient supervision is available for safety.

Dynamic Sitting Balance

Dynamic sitting balance is determined by having the patient short sit as above and then actively reach for objects in different directions such as toward the floor, the sides, and to the rear. Can the patient propel a wheelchair or reach for a footrest while maintaining trunk balance? The clinician will observe if the patient can shift weight to reach for the object/target and then recover to a midline position without loss of balance.

Protective Extension Reactions

Does the patient exhibit protective extension reactions by reaching out to the support surface with the arms to break a fall and protect the head?

Primitive Reflexes and Reactions

Does Stimulation or Self-Initiated Patient Movements Elicit Stereotypic Motor Responses?

The patient's positioning in a wheelchair may be negatively affected by primitive reflex activity (Figures 3-4 and 3-5). Identify the stimulus that triggers an undesirable response and control the response using adaptive equipment if necessary. For example, if an obligatory asymmetric tonic neck reflex (ATNR)[18] causes the patient to assume an asymmetrical "fencing" posture every time the head rotates out of midline, consider a headrest with a side panel to block and discourage

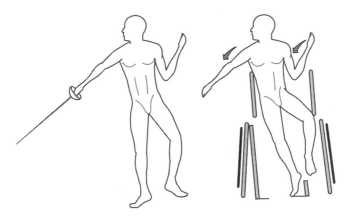

FIGURE 3-4 Patients who exhibit an ATNR assume a "fencing" posture and tend to place excessive pressure under one buttock in a wheelchair.

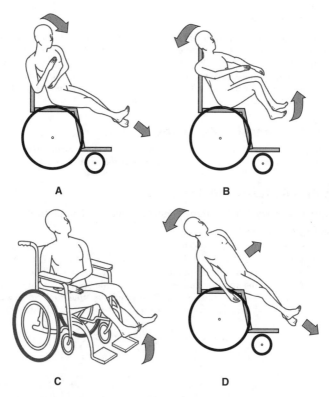

FIGURE 3-5 Primitive reflexes can indirectly affect pelvic position, resulting in forward sliding activity. **(A)** Symmetric tonic neck reflex (STNR), **(B)** STNR, **(C)** Negative support reaction, **(D)** tonic labyrinthine reflex (TLR).

head rotation to that side if tolerated while in the wheelchair. Note that primitive reflexes can indirectly affect pelvic position, resulting in forward sliding activity.

Asymmetric Tonic Neck Reflex (ATNR)—Head Rotation Can Result In (Figure 3-4):

- Limb extension and trunk convexity on the side of head rotation[18]
- Asymmetrical sitting—promotes a scoliotic posture
- Excessive asymmetrical weight bearing with risk of ulceration over an ischium or hip

Symmetric Tonic Neck Reflex (STNR)—Head Flexion/Extension Can Result In:
- LE extension with UE flexion when head flexes[18] (Figure 3-5A)
- LE flexion with UE extension when head extends[18] (Figure 3-5B)
- Forward sliding in wheelchair
- Sacral sitting with risk of sacral/coccyx ulceration

Supine Tonic Labyrinthine Reflex (TLR)—Reclined Position Can Result In (Figure 3-5D):
- Extension of trunk and extremities[18]
- Forward sliding in wheelchair
- Sacral sitting with risk of sacral/coccyx ulceration

Some patients may exhibit a supine TRL when reclined in a wheelchair, eliciting a strong extensor pattern in the trunk and extremities. These patients tend to "pop out" of their wheelchair and demonstrate forward sliding behavior. If present, such behavior would be an argument against recommending a recliner wheelchair.

Moro Reflex and Startle Reflex—Sudden Head Extension or Loud Noise Can Result In:
- Alternating extension-flexion extremity movements[18]
- Forward sliding in wheelchair

Positive Support Reaction—Foot Stimulation Can Result In:
- Strong extension of lower extremities[18]
- Extending, standing on, and possibly bending front rigging.

Negative Support Reaction—Foot Stimulation Can Result In (Figure 3-5C):
- Strong flexion of lower extremities[18]
- Posterior pelvic posture
- Sliding, sacral sitting with risk of sacral/coccyx ulceration
- Feet not remaining on footplates

Patients who exhibit a negative support reaction may tend to withdraw their LEs into flexion when their feet contact the front rigging. These patients may have difficulty resting their feet on the footplates. In addition, hyperflexion at the hips may pull on the hamstrings and result in posterior tilting of the pelvis and sacral sitting.

Muscle Tone

Normally, muscle tone, the readiness of muscle to move, will change according to the demands of a task. Clinicians should be concerned when muscle tone becomes inappropriately high, low, persistent, or fluctuating to the point that it interferes with the patient's function. Evaluate the patient under different gravitational conditions and joint position[5,8] such as upright sitting, supine, reclined sitting, backward tilted and sitting with hips flexed and abducted, to determine the effect of tone on patient alignment and ability to function. This can give you an idea of how to optimally position your patient in the wheelchair. Note that a patient may exhibit high tone in some body parts (e.g., limbs) and low tone in other areas (e.g., trunk) as is sometimes the case in CP spastic quadriplegia.

If Muscle Tone Is Excessively High

A patient with excessively high muscle tone may have difficulty relaxing into the seat of the wheelchair. Patients with excessively high tone tend to be rough on wheelchairs and can wear, bend, or break wheelchair components. Consider reinforcing wheelchair components (i.e., stronger hardware) that have been broken previously due to patient force. (I've seen several patients with severe neck extensor tone repeatedly destroy headrests.) Try to position patients so excessive tone is reduced; for example, excessive lower extremity extensor tone may be reduced if the patient's hips are positioned in flexion with abduction while sitting. A wide pommel placed between the knees can then help maintain this tone-reducing position.

If Muscle Tone Is Excessively Low

Patients with low tone have the feel of a Raggedy Anne doll when passively moved and may collapse their trunk into gravity while sitting upright. These patients are very difficult to support in an upright position and may require gravity-assisted sitting using a tilt or a reclined wheelchair frame.

If Muscle Tone Fluctuates

If tone changes from high to low, the constant movements associated with the tone changes may result in subtle or not so subtle pelvic movements and eventual sliding problems. Try to adequately stabilize the patient's pelvis with a seat belt secured across the hips to control patient sliding.

Muscle Tone Summary

If the patient has:

- *High flexor tone*—Trunk may pitch forward or knees may raise up toward the chest while in wheelchair.
- *High extensor tone*—Pelvis may thrust forward and patient may tend to stand up in wheelchair; frame or front rigging may break or bend.
- *Low tone*—Trunk may collapse into flexion.
- *Fluctuating tone*—Patient may tend to migrate and slide forward in wheelchair.
- *High tone secondary to spasticity*—Bumpy terrain may set off involuntary movement, altering the patient's position in the wheelchair relative to the control switch (joystick) and making operation of a power wheelchair difficult.[19]

Passive Range of Motion

Wheelchairs are generally designed for people who can flex their hip, knee, and ankle joints. In other words, to fit in a standard wheelchair, the patient must be able to bend their body into the shape of a chair.

Can Patients Flex Their Hips, Knees, and Ankles Sufficiently to Fit into a Standard Wheelchair?

Standard wheelchairs require standard positioning; that is, patients should possess at least 90 degrees of hip flexion, a 70-degree popliteal angle at the knee (i.e., –70 degrees of knee extension with hips in 90 degrees of flexion), and a neutral ankle position. If the patient is placed in a standard frame but lacks sufficient joint flexibility, particularly at the hips, sacral sitting, forward sliding, and pressure ulcers can ensue.[2]

Check for Flexibility:
- 90 degrees of hip flexion
- 70-degree popliteal angles
- Neutral ankle dorsiflexion

To determine if the patient has sufficient range of motion to sit upright in a standard wheelchair, do the following:

Step 1

First place the patient in supine and *slowly* flex both hips in the direction of the chest with the knees flexed so the hamstring muscles are placed on slack.[1] *Carefully* watch when the coccyx lifts off the mat.* If both hips can flex to a 90-degree angle so the thighs are pointing toward the ceiling while the coccyx remains on the mat, then the patient can probably fit in a standard wheelchair seat (Figure 3-6A). You may need to test each leg separately because of unilateral joint limitations or to management of limb weight during the test. Also, you may first need to relax the patient to rule out the effects of muscle tension or hypertonicity.

If, however, the patient's coccyx lifts off the mat *before* the hips reach 90 degrees (while the knees are flexed), then hip flexibility is probably inadequate for a standard wheelchair (Figure 3-6B). A reclining wheelchair or a wheelchair with a seat-to-back angle adjusted to an angle greater than 90 degrees (using hardware) will probably be necessary. Placing a patient who has hip flexion restrictions into a standard wheelchair will cause the patient to sacral sit and slide forward in the wheelchair. In my experience, limited hip mobility is a common cause of poor wheelchair positioning, often witnessed in nursing homes or when a generic wheelchair is shared among several patients.

---

* Alternatively, you can palpate over the patient's anterior superior iliac spine or observe for any changes in the neutral position of the patient's pelvis/low back in an effort to monitor for any undesirable pelvic or spinal motion during hip flexion.

CLINICAL EXAMINATION

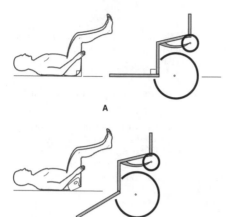

A

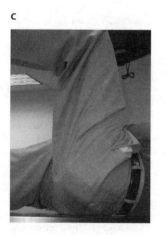

B

FIGURE 3-6 (A, C) Patients need 90 degrees of hip flexion to fit into a standard wheelchair. **(B, D)** A patient who exhibits less than 90-degrees of hip flexion will not have sufficient flexibility to sit upright in a standard frame and will need either a reclining frame or an open seat-to-back wheelchair angle (i.e., greater than 90 degrees).

C

D

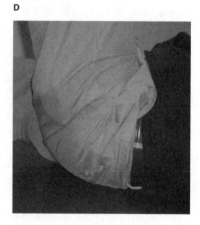

Step 2

Next determine if the patient has sufficient hamstring length to use standard 70-degree front rigging. In supine, with the patient's hips maintained in 90 degrees of flexion (if available), slowly extend both knees so the legs make a 70-degree angle with the vertical (i.e., 70-degree popliteal angles). (In this position, the fibula makes a 110-degree angle with the femur.) You may need to range each knee separately (Figure 3-7B).

If knee flexion contractures or hamstring tightness are present and the knees cannot be extended with the hips flexed, then the feet may need to be positioned with 90-degree front rigging or even underneath the wheelchair if tightness is extreme (Figure 3-7A and C). On the other hand, if knee *extension contractures* are present and the knees can extend but not flex, then an elevating leg rest may be needed to support the legs in extension.

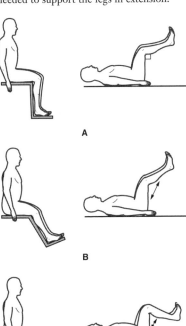

FIGURE 3-7 (A) Patients with tight hamstrings, exhibiting only 90-degree popliteal angles, may need to have their knees positioned with 90-degree front rigging. **(B)** Patients who have adequate hamstring length, exhibiting 70-degree popliteal angles, may be able to use standard front rigging in a wheelchair. **(C)** Patients who exhibit less than 90-degree popliteal angles may need their knees positioned in flexion with their feet supported underneath the wheelchair.

A

B

C

Step 3

Finally, check if the ankles can be dorsiflexed to a right angle when the knees are flexed. If the ankles are able to bend so the foot can rest flat on a surface, then a standard set of footplates may be adequate. If, however, an equinus deformity is present, then footplates with angle-adjustable capability may be needed (Figure 3-8).

Are Hip Abduction, Neutral Hip Rotation, and Neutral Subtalar Positions Possible in Sitting?

Correct to neutral if flexible; accommodate if deformities are fixed.

- *Hip adduction contractures*—May narrow the patient's sitting base and increase instability
- *Wind-swept hip position*—May require a wider frame because widest seat width measurements are now recorded from one hip to the contralateral knee (Figure 3-9)
- *Inverted and everted foot positions*—May cause excessive pressure over the lateral or medial border of the foot, respectively

Is UE Range of Motion Sufficient to Self-Propel a Wheelchair?

- Wrist flexion contractures limit the ability to grasp rear handrims.
- Elbow flexion contractures[20] restrict reach to rear wheels and forward wheelchair propulsion.
- Frozen shoulders may interfere with the propulsion and recovery phases of handrim propulsion.

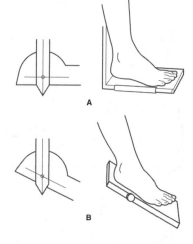

FIGURE 3-8 (A) Patients with neutral ankle range of motion may be supported by standard footplates. **(B)** Patients with a fixed equinus deformity may need adjustable footplates to accommodate the ankle joint restriction.

A

B

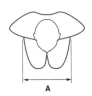
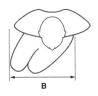

FIGURE 3-9 (A) Patient is symmetric and seat width is based on distance from hip to hip. **(B)** Patient with a fixed windswept deformity sitting with one hip adducted and the other hip abducted may need a wider seat.

A B

Is the Spine Straight and Flexible?

Determine if the patient's trunk is flexible or fixed by visually inspecting alignment or applying gentle tension to the spine. (See also Postural Alignment.)

First Approach: Evaluate Trunk Alignment*

While the patient is in supported sitting or supine on the mat, level the pelvis so that both anterior superior iliac spine (ASIS) landmarks are on the horizontal plane. Then, with the pelvis maintained in this level position, try to gently level the shoulders so that both acromial processes are also on a horizontal plane. If a level shoulder position cannot be attained, the spine may not be flexible enough to permit a symmetrical sitting. If an optimal symmetrical posture cannot be attained, try to at least balance the patient's head in midline over the patient's support base. A molded back insert can accommodate a fixed severe spinal deformity in a wheelchair.

Second Approach: Apply Tension to Spine

You may also assess spinal flexibility by applying gentle tension to the spine while the patient is sitting by gently leaning the patient forward. Check if the patient's back looks symmetrical or if there is a rib hump or hollow area on either side.

If the spine is not straight or if the back does not appear symmetric, refer the patient for orthopedic evaluation to rule out scoliosis. The referral is particularly important if the patient is still young and growing because the risk of curve progression is greater in this population.

Third Approach: Evaluation with a Clear Chair Back

Holmes et al., in their biomechanical study for managing neuromuscular scoliosis in persons with nonambulatory spastic cerebral palsy, suggested use of an evaluation chair with a *clear plastic back* so spinous processes can be visualized during attempts to correct alignment.[9]

---

* It may be useful to evaluate trunk alignment in three planes: frontal, transverse, and sagittal. (See Exercise 1 at the end of this chapter.)

Skin

Is Skin Intact?

Skin is our body's first line of defense against infection. With the patient's permission, inspect all bony areas of the body that are at risk of pressure ulcer development from prolonged or excessive weight bearing while sitting. Red areas that remain visible for more than 30 minutes are at risk for skin breakdown and should be relieved from pressure until normal skin color returns.[13]* It is critical to actually inspect at-risk areas like the ischium rather than accept a caregiver's description. An aide once reported a little sore on her client; when I visually inspected the area with the patient in sidelying, I saw a hole the size of my fist.

Inspect for:

- Breaks in skin
- Red coloration
- Bruises
- Scars
- Old, healed pressure sore areas
- Graft sites[20]

Vulnerable areas

Bony weight-bearing areas:

- Ischia
- Coccyx
- Greater trochanters
- Spinous processes
- Scapula
- Ears
- Back of head
- Elbows
- Knees
- Ankles/heels

Risk Factors for Pressure Ulcers[21]

- Diagnosis
- UE function
- Postural deformity
- Number of hours in wheelchair
- Types of activities
- Terrain

---

* This is probably only a rough guideline.

- Temperature
- Mosture, perspiration, drainage from wound[22]
- Level of inactivity or independence
- History of tissue compromises
- Incontinence
- Sitting pressures (compression and shear duration, intensity)[22] and distribution
- Body build—thin patients[23]
- Malnutrition[22]
- Chronic disease (Alzheimer's, diabetes mellitus)[22]
- Medications (sedatives, tranquilizers, steroids, cytotoxics)[22]
- Cigarette smoking, drug abuse, alcohol[22]
- Psychological (self-esteem,[22] depression[24])
- Dehydration[22]
- Perspiration

Cushion Wear: Clues to Weight Bearing in Sitting

Seat cushion wear may hint to how the patient habitually sits in his or her wheelchair. If patients sit properly, the seat may eventually wear symmetrically at the rear of the seat. If the front of the seat is worn, it suggests the patient slides forward and may be placing weight on his or her sacrum in the wheelchair. If the cushion is worn on one side, it may suggest the patient is sitting asymmetrically with excessive pressure over one ischium and trochanter (Figure 3-10). Suspected skin areas can be further assessed.

- *Seat worn in front*—Patient sliding forward
- *Seat worn on one side*—Patient sitting asymmetrically
- *Seat worn in center rear*—Patient sitting in the center

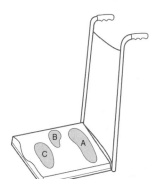

FIGURE 3-10 A worn seat can suggest where the patient habitually sits on the cushion. **(A)** Wear in center rear of cushion. **(B)** Wear on one side suggests asymmetrical sitting over one hip. **(C)** Wear in front suggests sliding activity and possible sacral sitting.

Assessment Tools

Risk Assessment Scales

Risk assessment scales offer an estimate (but not a certainty) of pressure ulcer risk. Using meta-analysis, Pancorbo-Hidalgo et al. found the Braden scale to be a good risk predictor (odds ratio = 4.08, CI 95% = 2.56–6.48; sensitivity 57.1%; specificity 67.5%) and the Norton Scale a "reasonable" risk predictor (OR = 2.16, CI 95% = 1.03–4.54; sensitivity 46.8%; specificity 61.8%) for pressure ulcers.[25] Interestingly, clinical judgment of nurses was not a good predictor.*

Pressure Mapping

Pressure mapping may be a useful tool for evaluating weight-bearing pressures under the ischium, and can assist in cushion selection for a particular patient.

Pressure mapping involves using a set of sensors (a mat) between the seat surface and the buttocks to record and display pressure levels at the patient's seat/skin interface (Figure 3-11).

Advantages

These data can offer the following benefits:

- *Identify peak pressures*—Determine the peak pressures and distribution of pressures occurring between a particular patient's buttocks and seat cushion.
- *Uncover problem pressure areas*—Determine the presence of excessive weight-bearing areas not detected during a postural and skin exam.[26]
- *Develop pressure relief strategies*—Determine the type of pressure relief strategy that works best for a *particular* patient (e.g., frame tilt or recline, wheelchair push-up, rolling/leaning, and to what extent). For example, how far does the patient need to lean forward on a particular cushion in order to relieve pressure under the ischia.[26]

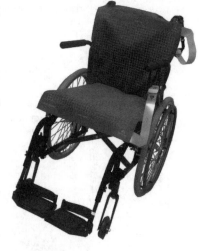

FIGURE 3-11 Pressure mapping technology (Photo Courtesy of Tecksan, Inc.).

---

* Small sample; $n = 3$

- *Patient-specific cushion comparisons*—Determine which cushion of several evaluated offers the lowest peak pressures under the ischia for a *particular* patient.[26,27]
- *Seat pressure education*—Helpful in educating and illustrating how a patient's sitting behavior affects pressure conditions in the wheelchair.
- *Funding justification*—Offers some evidence for the medical justification of a particular cushion that was evaluated (e.g., cushion offered the lowest peak pressure values under the ischia of all cushions tested with this patient).[26]

Limitations

Pressure mapping also has several limitations:

- *Apples and oranges comparison*—Pressure mapping may be misleading when comparing cushion studies employing different methodologies; that is, different studies using different methodologies and measuring devices may have cushion outcomes that are just not comparable.[22]
- *Within group variability*—A great deal of individual differences exists for pressure outcomes, even within the same diagnostic population. Garber et al.[28] assessed bony and soft tissue sitting pressures in 57 patients (mostly SCI tetraplegia/paraplegia) while sitting on six different cushions (foam, air, and flotation).[28] Although they found some cushions provided lower pressures than others, there was no "universal cushion" that could be recommended for their study group, purported to be similar. For any given person in the study, outcomes varied, with some cushions providing good relief under bone, and other cushions offering poor relief. The authors argued against an "uncritical prescription" for an entire class of patients.
- *Generalizability problem*—It is probably misleading to generalize pressure mapping data generated from nondisabled people to a patient population. Hobson, for example, reported that average maximal seating pressures measured 1.5 to 2.5 times higher in complete but active SCI wheelchair users ($n = 12$; 5 tetraplegia; 7 paraplegia; age 25–66 years) as compared with a nondisabled group ($n = 10$; age 28–57) using similar methodology.[29]
- *Insensitivity to deep tissue*—Pressure mapping only provides information on interface pressures at the skin/cushion interface. There is evidence that pressure ulcers not only originate superficially and progress more deeply, but also originate deeply, at the muscle/bone level, and progress superficially.[22] Pressure mapping cannot directly measure these deeper pressure levels.
- *Questioning the 32 mm Hg threshold*—The traditional guideline of staying below an interface pressure of 32 mm Hg to stave off pressure ulcer risk may be misguided. The 32 mm Hg cutoff point was based on healthy subject data (on nail beds) and may not be a true reflection of actual capillary pressures under the buttocks in persons with real health problems. Clinically important values may be higher or lower than this value.[30,31]
- *Other considerations*—Beyond interface pressures, additional cushion considerations include temperature and moisture control, weight and stability

characteristics, cost/benefit ratios (i.e., evidence-based effectiveness keeping costs in mind), maintenance and monitoring requirements, and service and warrantees.

Relieving Pressure

Provide at-risk areas with pressure reduction by removing the offending local pressure source or distributing the force over a greater surface area.

- Shape the support surface.
- Use static pressure-reducing seat cushion materials (foams, air, gel).
- Use dynamic seating (power-operated).
- Use a recliner or tilt-in-space frame to alter weight-bearing areas (a 65-degree tilt angle may be required).[32]
- Teach active weight shifting in wheelchair to the patient. Be aware that sitting push-ups require UE strength; lateral trunk bending/rolling from side to side requires less UE strength but greater trunk control.[32,33]
- Instruct caregivers to periodically lift the patient from the seat surface to relieve the continuous source of pressure.
- Alter risk factors (i.e., terrain, nutrition, climate, hours sitting, activity level).

Weight-Shifting Strategies

Lateral shifting, forward leaning, backward tilting, and reclining can lower pressure levels during wheelchair sitting. Hobson reported maximal pressure reduction up to 38% during 15-degree lateral trunk bending (on unweighted side), 9% during 50-degree forward flexion, 12% during 120-degree recline, and 11% during a 20-degree backward tilt in complete but active SCI wheelchair users ($n = 12$; 5 tetraplegia; 7 paraplegia; age 25–66 years).[29] Although the recline position led to a reduction in peak pressure, 120- and 110-degree recline also led to a 25% and 7% rise in shear, respectively. On the other hand, Hobson estimated a 25-degree backward tilt would reduce shear to about zero.

Weight-Shifting Durations

The time required to recover from sitting pressures may be longer than the customary 15–30 seconds. In a retrospective chart review of 46 new and chronic SCI patients (19 tetraplegia, 27 paraplegia) who attended a seating clinic, Coggrave and Rose reported that the time required to raise tissue oxygen levels to unloaded levels ranged from 42 seconds to 3 minutes, 30 seconds (average 1 minute, 51 seconds).[32] This finding questions the conventional guideline that 15–30 seconds is sufficient time to recover from weight bearing. It further suggests these longer durations to unload pressure by performing a sitting push-up may be too taxing on the UEs, particularly if the patient has preexisting shoulder pathology.

Are There Lumps, Bumps, or Bruises?

Skin markings can suggest rubbing or a repeatedly injured body part. Lumps can suggest inflammation, cysts, or tumors. Check for callouses on the knees or elbows for indications of excessive weight bearing in these areas. Check for bruising on the upper or lower limbs resulting from banging into metal or hard wheelchair components. Check for masses (cysts) on or below the skin that may require pressure relief in the seating system. Refer questionable masses for medical evaluation. Report suspected signs of child abuse to the appropriate agency.

- *Calloused areas*—Provide pressure relief.
- *Bruised areas*—Provide padding.
- *Prominent bony areas*—Cut out a pressure relief area.
- *Masses*—Refer for medical evaluation.
- *Suspicious signs of child abuse*—Report to appropriate state agency.

Sensation

Does the Patient Report Discomfort When Sitting?

If yes, the good news is that the patient is probably sensate and capable of feeling pain. Pain is an important warning signal that tissue damage may be occurring. The ability to adjust position due to discomfort is dependent on intact sensation.[20]

Pain sensation can be tested using a sterile disposable safety pin and asking the patient to report sharp and dull.[34] Please note the patient may still retain touch sensation and yet be anesthetic to pain because separate neurotracts can mediate these two modalities. Examine anesthetic areas on the patient that contact the back and seat for signs of impending pressure ulcers.

Measuring Discomfort

Crane et al. describe a self-reported seating discomfort assessment tool, called the Wheelchair Seating Discomfort Assessment Tool (WcS-DAT), designed to quantify sitting discomfort in long-term, active wheelchair users who have sensation.[35] The tool includes sections on wheelchair-related discomfort issues, questions regarding discomfort resulting in a general discomfort score (GDS), and body areas involved leading to a discomfort intensity score (DIS). In a group of 28 multiple sclerosis (MS), amyotrophic lateral sclerosis (ALS), post-polio syndrome, and muscular dystrophy (MD) wheelchair users (n = 17 to 27) who sat more than 8 hours a day, test retest reliability (ICCs) for 1-hour or 1-week intervals ranged from 0.83 to 0.97. Concurrent validity ranged from r = –0.024 to 0.92 for comfort and discomfort items on the chair evaluation checklist (CEC) and from 0.70 to 0.93 for items on the Short Form McGill Pain Questionnaire (SF-MPQ).

Does the Patient Experience Pain?

Although pain is a useful warning sign for impending tissue damage, it can also interfere with function. Manual wheelchair use, for example, has been associated with various UE pain-related pathologies that, in turn, can interfere with the ability to self-propel handrim wheelchairs.

In a self-reported survey of 92 persons with tetraplegia and 103 persons with paraplegia (28% response rate) who were a minimum of 1 year since injury and who used a manual wheelchair at least 3 hours/week, 78% of the tetraplegic and 59% of the paraplegic sample reported having experienced shoulder pain since receiving their wheelchair.[36] Boninger et al. found that median nerve function was associated with rapid loading of the pushrims during propulsion in 34 persons with paraplegia, suggesting a possible greater risk of developing median nerve injuries using this loading pattern.[37] Mercer et al. found that shoulder joint force levels occurring during handrim propulsion were associated with shoulder pathology (i.e., edema, thickening) detected on MRI in 33 persons with paraplegia.[38,39]

Measuring Pain

Shoulder pain is common in persons with SCI, so it would be useful to quantify it. Curtis et al. developed a Wheelchair User's Shoulder Pain Index (WUSPI) to measure shoulder pain using a functional 15-item self-reporting questionnaire for long-term wheelchair users (majority SCI).[40] Test retest reliability and validity (WUSPI scores with shoulder extension, flexion, abduction ROM scores) were excellent (ICC 0.99) and fair ($r = -0.30$ to -0.48), respectively, for activities involving wheelchair propulsion, dressing, transfer, and general activities.

Is Position Sense Diminished in the Limbs?

Position sense (i.e., the ability to know the location of a limb in space without vision) is important for motor control.[41] Position sense can be tested by having the patient attempt to reproduce a passively displaced limb position without the aid of vision. If the patient lacks position sense of a limb, he or she may need to rely on vision to perform motor tasks like propelling the wheels, operating the wheel locks, or adjusting the footrest. Patients may also have difficulty operating a proportional joystick control for power mobility if UE proprioception is involved. If vision is necessary to compensate for diminished position sense, make sure the patient's vision is not obstructed by equipment.

Is Vision or Hearing Impaired?

Visual problems will significantly limit independent self-mobility because the patient will not see where he or she is going. Consider referral for an eye evaluation and possible eyeglasses to improve vision. If the patient has diminished hearing, warning sounds such as sirens, conversation, and instructional efforts may not be appreciated and the patient may feel isolated. Consider a referral for an auditory evaluation and possible hearing aids.

Screen For

- Blindness
- Peripheral vision deficits
- Hemianopsia—field cuts
- Hearing impairment

Speed/Endurance

Can Functional Distances Be Achieved in a Reasonable Time?

Functional distance is a relative measure and depends on where the patient needs to go and when he or she wants to get there. How far can the patient propel a wheelchair? Is this a meaningful distance for the patient in his or her particular neighborhood (i.e., getting to work, to the bus, to the store, into an elevator, crossing a street)? Reporting that the patient can propel 150 feet is not as meaningful as stating that the patient can propel 150 feet to the corner drug store and back within 15 minutes without help. Measure how many feet the client can self-propel to a destination and how many minutes it takes to reach the destination. *Even timed tasks within the patient's home are important because Medicare bases wheelchair funding decisions, in part, on a patient's ability to finish a mobility-related activity of daily living (ADL) in a reasonable time period (see Appendix A).*[42] If endurance is limited or the patient is a marginal wheelchair user, a lighter weight frame or power mobility may be justifiable.

Speed can give an indication of how mobile nursing residents will be in wheelchairs. In a 2-day observational study of 65 nonambulatory, cognitively involved nursing home residents (mean age 85; mean MMSE 9.8), Simmons et al. found that speed of propulsion was a predictor for the amount of time residents were observed propelling around the residence in the wheelchair (multiple $r = 0.45$, $p < 0.02$).[43]

Strength

Does the Patient Have Sufficient Muscle Strength to Perform Wheelchair Skills?

Patients need enough strength to disengage wheel locks, manage front rigging, and propel a wheelchair (e.g., up an incline). In fact, a patient who cannot disengage wheel locks in order to propel will have limited independence.[43] Most skills performed against gravity require muscle grades to be *greater than fair*.

Is Adequate Strength Available in the Upper Limbs

- To shift body weight sideways to perform a pressure-relieving push-up?
- To propel the wheels?
- To stop the wheelchair?
- To engage the wheel locks?
- To lift a front rigging or armrest?

Is Strength Adequate in the Lower Limbs

- To propel the wheelchair with the feet?
- To lift the foot onto the footplate?
- To assist in transfers out of the wheelchair?

Strength and Handrim Propulsion

Although strength may correlate with the forces applied to a handrim, it does not necessarily mean the patient will be efficient at wheelchair propulsion. In an observational study involving 22 persons with SCI (T2–L1; 16 men, 6 women; ages 43 ± 9.5; years with diagnosis 16.6 ± 7.4), Ambrosio et al. found that shoulder isokinetic peak torques failed to correlate with productive wheel motion, that is, pushrim cadence or fraction of effective force (FEF)[44] (where FEF = Ft^2/FR is the tangential handrim force that permits forward wheel motion, squared, divided by total resultant handrim force).

Strength Versus Spasticity

Spasticity, although not a measure of muscle strength, is sometimes harnessed by patients to perform skills such as adjusting sitting posture or transferring out of a wheelchair.

Cognition

Does the Patient Exhibit Intentional Behavior?

Means-end behavior, or the ability to use a means to achieve an end, is normally attained within the first 2 years of development[45] (Piaget's sensorimotor period). An example of this behavior is pulling on a string to acquire a toy. Acquisition of this behavior is required to intentionally act on the environment and problem solve. One also needs intentional behavior to operate manual and power mobility.

Cognition and Power Mobility

Problem solving may be an important indicator for power chair readiness. Furumasu et al. found that the score on a Pediatric Powered Wheelchair Screening

Test (PPWST), a cognitive assessment battery that tests problem solving and spatial relations, predicted (explaining 74% of the variance) overall power wheelchair readiness in 15 children with cerebral palsy who used a joystick and were not profoundly developmentally delayed.[46]

Cognition is also an important factor when recommending power mobility for children. In a national survey of pediatric power wheelchair providers (46% suppliers and 54% clinicians [PT/OT] with a response rate of 37%), Guerette et al. found 41% of respondents did not recommend power mobility for a child because of limited cognition.[47] Concerns included a lack of understanding of the control mechanisms (cause-effect understanding), an inability to negotiate around an obstacle (problem-solving ability), and distractibility.

Perception

Do Perceptual Deficits Affect Wheelchair Safety?

- *Spatial relations and power mobility*—Along with cognition, spatial relations ability is a predictor for power wheelchair readiness in children with CP.[46]
- *Unilateral (hemispatial) neglect*—Does the patient bump into objects and people on one side of the environment[48] or consistently turn the wheelchair in one direction only? In a replication study, Webster et al. confirmed previous findings that right CVA patients ($n = 25$) with hemi neglect as determined by a letter cancellation test (LCT) ran directly into and left sideswiped more objects while on a wheelchair obstacle course than right CVA patients without hemi neglect or left CVA patients.[49]
- *Depth perception*—Is depth misjudged[48] (i.e., stairs, curbs, and architectural barriers)?
- *Figure ground*—Can foreground (people, obstacles) be distinguished from background?[48]

Motivation

Is the Patient Motivated to Operate a Wheelchair?

A patient's power wheelchair may end up in a closet, never to be used if the patient was never motivated to use it in the first place. In fact, Medicare wants to know if the patient is on board with the recommendation (that is, compliant) before a wheelchair request is funded.[42] Provide a sufficient trial period to determine if equipment will be used by the patient.

- *Motivated*—Encourage independence if safe.
- *Unmotivated*—Provide a sufficient trial period; reevaluate goals; refer to psychologist if patient appears depressed.

CLINICAL EXAMINATION

Judgment

Is Judgment Adequate for Safe Wheelchair Use?

If the patient is motivated but lacks judgment, catastrophe can ensue. A wheelchair provides mobility, which can bring the patient closer to a danger such as thermal sources in a kitchen, stairwells in a building, or oncoming traffic at an intersection. Assess judgment under real-life condition with the wheelchair.

- *Good judgment*—Encourage independent mobility.
- *Poor judgment*—Limited independence[50]; encourage safe, supervised, or limited mobility. Keep away from stairways and roadways.

Memory

Patients with memory deficits may fail to remember basic wheelchair safety procedures such as engaging wheel locks before transferring into or out of their wheelchair. These patients may also get lost if traveling alone and therefore require supervision.

Poor Memory

- Encourage supervised mobility.[50]
- Provide identification for patient and wheelchair.

Vital Functions

Is Orthostatic Hypotension Present?

A patient may not be able to tolerate upright sitting or transfer into a wheelchair safely if bouts of dizziness occur as a result of a drop in blood pressure. Measure blood pressure changes from lying to sitting. If a drop in systolic pressure greater than 20 mm Hg occurs upon sitting up, consider the following strategies:

- Gradually change positions
- Use a reclining back or backward tilting frame to enable the head of the patient to be lowered as needed to improve sitting tolerance.
- Refer for medical evaluation.

General and Local Body Shape

Consider body shape issues that may affect wheelchair selection (see Appendix E).[51,52]

EXERCISES

1. a. Try to view your friend's body segment three-dimensionally. For example, for the shoulders, determine whether they are level or if one side is higher or lower when *viewed from the front*. Next, determine if the shoulders both face front or if one is rotated more forward or backward when *viewed from above (aerial view)*. Finally, determine if the shoulders are aligned over the hips or are instead leaning too far forward when *viewed from the side*.
   b. Repeat this exercise with the pelvis. These exercises can be done with most body parts to determine how symmetric or balanced body segments are in space.
2. What are the critical ROM ranges at the hip, knee, and ankle needed to fit into a standard wheelchair?
3. Name at least five risk factors for developing a pressure ulcer.
4. How would you define "ideal posture"?
5. Is it more important to have a large amount or a reliable amount of movement to operate the controls of a power wheelchair?
6. What basic anthropometric measurements are needed to prescribe a frame size?
7. Practice taking anthropometric measurements on a friend in both the sitting and supine position. How did measurements of back height and seat width in the two positions compare?
8. How would patients with either high or low muscle tone influence your wheelchair prescription?
9. Would a custom molded back insert be appropriate for a patient who has a functional scoliosis that is flexible and correctable to neutral?
10. What is the most hazardous environmental factor related to wheelchair-related deaths?
11. Your patient assumes a persistent fencing posture while sitting in a wheelchair. What pathological reflex causes this posturing and what positioning problems are associated with it?

References

1. Bergen AF, Presperin J, Tallman T. *Positioning for Function: Wheelchairs and Other Assistive technologies*. Valhalla, NY: Valhalla Rehabilitation; 1990:13–82.
2. Kamenetz HL. *The Wheelchair Book: Mobility for the Disabled*. Springfield, CT: Charles C Thomas; 1969:128–134.
3. Delisa JA, Greenberg S. Wheelchair prescription guidelines. *Am Fam Physician*. 1982:24:145–150.
4. Brubaker C. Ergonometric considerations. *J Rehabil Res Dev*. 1990;2(Supp):37–48.
5. Feldenkrais M. *Body and Mature Behavior: A Study of Anxiety, Sex, Gravitation, and Learning*. New York: New York International University Press; 1949:68.

CLINICAL EXAMINATION

6. Sprigle S, Wootten M, Sawacha Z, Thielman G. Relationships among cushion type, backrest height, seated posture, and reach of wheelchair users with spinal cord injury [erratum]. *J Spinal Cord Med*. 2004;27(3):262.

7. Bolin I, Bodin P, Kreuter M. Sitting position—posture and performance in C5–C6 tetraplegia. *Spinal Cord*. 2000;38:425–434.

8. Taylor SJ. An overview of evaluation for wheelchair seating for people who have had strokes. (Innovations in practice.) *Top Stroke Rehabil*. 2003;10(1):95–99.

9. Holmes KJ, Michael SM, Thorpe SL, Solomonidis SE. Management of scoliosis with special seating for the non-ambulant spastic cerebral palsy population—a biomechanical study. *Clin Biomech*. 2003;18:480–487.

10. Taylor SJ. Evaluating the client with physical disabilities for wheelchair sitting. *Am J Occup Ther*. 1987;41:711–716.

11. Grunewald J. Wheelchair selection from a nursing perspective. *Rehabil Nurs*. 1986;11:31–32.

12. Currie DM, Hardwick K, Marburger RA, Britell CW. Wheelchair prescription and adaptive seating. In Delisa JL, Gans BM, eds. *Rehabilitation Medicine: Principles and Practice*, 2nd ed. Philadelphia: JB Lippincott; 1993:563–585.

13. Donovan WH, Dinh TA, Garber SL, Krouskop TA, Rodriguez GP, Shenaq SM. Pressure ulcers. In Delisa JL, Gans BM, eds. *Rehabilitation Medicine: Principles and Practice*, 2nd ed. Philadelphia: JB Lippincott; 1993:716–732.

14. Warren CG. Technical considerations: power mobility and its implications. *J Rehabil Res Dev*. 1990;2(Supp):74–85.

15. Panel for the Prediction and Prevention of Pressure Ulcers in Adults. *Pressure Ulcers in Adults: Prediction and Prevention. Clinical Practice Guideline, Number 3*. AHCPR Pub No. 92-0047. Rockville, MD: Agency for Health Care Policy and Research, Public Health Service, U.S. Department of Health and Human Services; May 1992:5.

16. Calder CJ, Kirby RL. Fatal wheelchair-related accidents in the United States. *Am J Phys Med Rehabil*. 1990;69:184–190.

17. Ragnarsson KT. Clinical perspectives on wheelchair selection: prescription considerations and a comparison of conventional and light weight wheelchairs. *J Rehabil Res Dev*. 1990;2(Supp):8–16.

18. Fiorentino MR. *Reflex Testing Methods for Evaluating CNS Development*, 2nd ed. Springfield, IL: Charles C Thomas; 1981:14–21.

19. Ozer MN. Clinical perspectives on wheelchair selection: a participatory planning process for wheelchair selection. *J Rehabil Res Dev*. 1990;2(Supp):31–36.

20. Behrman AL. Clinical perspectives on wheelchair selection: factors in functional assessment. *J Rehabil Res Dev*. 1990;2(Supp):17–27.

21. Garber SL. Wheelchair cushions: a historical review. *Am J Occup Ther*. 1985;39:453–459.

22. Agam L, Gefen A. Pressure ulcers and deep tissue injury: a bioengineering perspective. 2007;16(8):336–342.

23. Garber SL, Krouskop TA. Body build and its relationship to pressure distribution in the seated wheelchair patient. *Arch Phys Med Rehabil*. 1982;63:17–20.

24. Smith BM, Guihan M, LaVela SL, Garber SL. Factors predicting pressure ulcers in veterans with spinal cord injuries. *Am J Phys Med Rehabil*. 2008;87(9):750–757.

25. Pancorbo-Hidalgo PL, Garcia-Fernandez FP, Lopez-Medina IM, Alvarez-Nieto C. Risk assessment scales for pressure ulcer prevention: a systematic review. *J Adv Nurs*. 2006;54(1):94–110.

26. Smith R. Devising a system. *Rehab Manage*. 2008;21(2):10, 12–15.

27. Brienza DM, Geyer MJ. Using support surfaces to manage tissue integrity advances in skin and wound care. *Adv Skin Wound Care*. 2005;18(3):151–157.

28. Garber SL, Krouskop TA, Carter RE. A system for clinically evaluating wheelchair pressure-relief cushions. *Am J Occup Ther*. 1978;32(9):565–570.

29. Hobson DA. Comparative effects of posture on pressure and shear at the body-seat interface. *J Rehabil Res Devel*. 1992;29(4):21–31.

30. Krouskop TA, Garber SL. Interface pressure measurements. *J Enterostomal Ther*. 1990;17(4):182.

31. Gefen A. The biomechanics of sitting-acquired pressure ulcers in patients with spinal cord injury or lesions. *Int Wound J*. 2007;4:222–231.

32. Coggrave MJ, Rose LS. A specialist seating assessment clinic: changing pressure relief practice. *Spinal Cord*. 2003;41:692–695.

33. Stockton L, Rithalia S. Is dynamic seating a modality worth considering in the prevention of pressure ulcers? *J Tissue Viability*. 2007;17:15–21.

34. Swartz MH. *Textbook of Physical Diagnosis: History and Examination*. Philadelphia: WB Saunders; 1989:506.

35. Crane BA, Holm MB, Hobson D, Cooper RA, Reed MP, Stadelmeier S. Test-retest, internal item consistency, and concurrent validity of the Wheelchair Seating Discomfort Assessment Tool. *Assist Technol*. 2005;17(2):98–107.

36. Curtis KA, Drysdale GA, Lanza RD, Kolber M, Vitolo RS, West R. Shoulder pain in wheelchair users with tetraplegia and paraplegia. *Arch Phys Med Rehabil*. 1999;80(4):453–457.

37. Boninger ML, Cooper RA, Baldwin MA, Shimada SD, Koontz A. Wheelchair pushrim kinetics: body weight and median nerve function. *Arch Phys Med Rehabil*. 1999;80:910–915.

38. Mercer JL, Boninger M, Koontz A, Ren D, Dyson-Hudson T, Cooper R. Shoulder joint kinetics and pathology in manual wheelchair users. *Clin Biomech*. 2006;21:781–789.

39. Levy CE, Chow JW. Pushrim-activated power-assist wheelchairs: elegance in motion. *Am J Phys Med Rehabil*. 2004;83(2):166-167.

40. Curtis KA, Roach KE, Applegate EB, et al. Reliability and validity of the wheelchair user's shoulder pain index (WUSPI). *Paraplegia*. 1995;33(10):595–601.

41. Magill RA. *Motor Learning: Concepts and Applications*. 4th ed. Madison, WI: WCB Brown & Benchmark; 1993:96.

42. Centers for Medicare and Medicaid Services. An algorithmic approach to determine if mobility assistive equipment is reasonable and necessary for medicare beneficiaries with a personal mobility deficit (CR3791—Mobility Assistive Equipment (MAE)). *MLN Matters*. 2005, June 3; MM3791. Available at: http://www.cms.hhs.gov/MLNMatters Articles/downloads/MM3791.pdf. Accessed January 15, 2008.

43. Simmons SF, Schnelle JF, MacRae PG, Ouslander JG. Wheelchair as mobility restraints: Predictors of wheelchair activities in nonambulatory nursing home residence. *J Am Geriatr Soc*. 1995;43(4):384–388.

44. Ambrosio F, Boninger ML, Souza AL, Fitzgerald SG, Koontz AM, Cooper RA. Biomechanics and strength of manual wheelchair users. *J Spinal Cord Med*. 2005;28(5):407–414.

45. Rosenblith JF, Sims-Knight JE. *In the Beginning: Development in the First Two Years*. Newbury Park, CA: Sage; 1989:411–415.

46. Furumasu J, Guerette P, Tefft D. Relevance of the pediatric powered wheelchair screening test for children with cerebral palsy. *Dev Med Child Neurol*. 2004; 46:468–474.

47. Guerette P, Tefft D, Furumasu J. Pediatric powered wheelchairs: results of a national survey of providers. *Asst Technol*. 2005;17:144–158.

CLINICAL EXAMINATION

48. Siev E, Freishtat B, Zoltan B. *Perceptual and Cognitive Dysfunction in the Adult Stroke Patient: A Manual for Evaluation and Treatment.* Rev ed. Thorofare, NJ: Slack; 1986:53–87.

49. Webster JS, Rapport LJ, Godlewski MC, Abadee PS. Effect of attentional bias to right space on wheelchair mobility. *J Clin Exp Neuropsychol.* 1994;16(1):129–137.

50. Mattingly D. Wheelchair selection. *Orthop Nurs.* 1993;12:11–17.

51. Sheldon WH. *The Varieties of Human Physique: An Introduction to Constitution Psychology.* New York: Harper & Brothers; 1940:1–9.

52. Tortora PG, Eubank K. *Survey of Historic Costume: A History of Western Dress,* 2nd ed. New York: Fairchild;1994:304–305.

CHAPTER 4

Functional Examination

Functional Examination

The functional examination is critical to consider when determining wheelchair needs and includes locomotion, transfers, sitting, and upper limb abilities.

The key question is: What can the patient do?

Locomotion

Does the Patient Need a Wheelchair?

If the patient is a functional ambulator, safely ambulates to required destinations without help (i.e., with or without assistive device and bracing), and can keep up with his or her peers, then a wheelchair is not needed. Consider a wheelchair if the patient cannot safely ambulate or if walking is limited to short distances.

If a Wheelchair is Needed, Can the Patient Self Propel a Manual Wheelchair?

If the patient cannot functionally walk, determine if self-propelling a manual wheelchair is possible using the upper or lower extremities.[1]

If the patient uses the upper extremities (UEs) to self-propel, adjust the rear wheel position to optimize propulsion efforts and consider a lower back insert to permit the upper trunk extension movements that occur during self-propulsion. If the patient uses the lower extremities (LEs) to self-propel, consider a low seat with the front of the seat beveled (undercut) so the back of the patient's knees do not hit the front edge of the seat as the feet pull under the wheelchair. Also remember that some patients may be more functional using their feet to propel the wheelchair backward rather than forward.

Tools to Assess Wheelchair Skills

In a systematic review from 1966 to 2001 (limited to English language speakers), Kilkens et al. identified 24 different wheelchair skills tests for handrim manual wheelchairs.[2] The most common assessed skills included propulsion; transfers;

curb, slope, and track negotiation; sprinting; and wheelies. Additional activities included obstacle courses, figure eights, and slalom. Most tests targeted spinal cord injury (SCI) populations and measured time, level of independence, physical strain, distance, and velocity. Of the 24 tests, only 10 tests reported validity, 9 reported reliability, and 3 reported sensitivity to change. The *wheelchair skills test (WST)* was the only instrument deemed to have sufficient validity and reliability. The authors recommend that only tests with adequate validity, reliability, and sensitivity should be used.

Subjective Estimation of Wheelchair Abilities

In a study that evaluated the validity between the objective wheelchair skills test (WST) and subjective estimates of ability in 21 individuals with amputations, strokes, musculoskeletal diagnoses, and SCI, patients overestimated their wheelchair abilities by almost 18%.[3] Estimates were generally accurate for wheel locks, footrest, door management, and wheelie operations. On the other hand, less accurate estimates were found for activities involving transfers, armrests, high object reaching, picking up objects from the floor, ascending inclines, and negotiating surfaces (small curbs, gravel, or irregular surfaces). Although rank correlations (Spearman) between subjective estimates and observations were excellent (0.95) to good (0.75) for patients and therapists, respectively, more accurate information on wheelchair skills can be obtained using objective (observable) testing.

If the Patient Cannot Self-Propel, Is Power Wheelchair Use Possible?

If the patient cannot functionally walk or self-propel a manual wheelchair, but may be safe and independent using a power wheelchair, consider an evaluation and trial for power mobility. Much thought must go into a power wheelchair recommendation because the patient's community (i.e., home, streets, school, bus, stores) must be accessible and the power wheelchair will require upkeep.

Power Mobility Evaluations

The patient should be evaluated *in* a power chair. They should be evaluated for (1) postural support system, (2) type of mobility base, and (3) type of controls. Judgment (stop at corners, driveways, and crossways), perception, means-ends behavior (cause and effect), and some reliable movement to operate the controls are required. The patient needs to stop when required, slow down near doors, and look left and right to avoid hazards.[4] Determine if the patient can safely negotiate straight paths, turns, elevators, door openings, crowds, and outdoor terrain. Additional indoor/outdoor driving skills to evaluate include the ability to follow directions, understand directionality, recognize/avoid obstacles or danger (adequate vision/problem solving), and access/activate control switches under varying terrain conditions and during public transportation.[5]

Predictors of Power Wheelchair Performance

In children, Furumasu et al. found that scores on a Pediatric Powered Wheelchair Screening Test (PPWST), a cognitive assessment battery that tests problem solving and spatial relations, predicted (74% of the variance) overall power wheelchair readiness in 15 children with cerebral palsy who used a joystick and were not profoundly developmentally delayed.[6]

In adults, Massengale et al. found that driving performance with a power chair, using the Power Mobility Road Test, was related to patients' visual perception ($r = 0.59$), ocular motor function (saccades, pursuits, $r = 0.44$–0.60), stereo-depth perception ($r = 0.42$), far binocular vision ($r = 0.35$), environmental alertness (picture completion, $r = 0.42$), and possession of a drivers license ($r = 0.45$).[7]*

If None of the Above Works, Consider Attendant Assistance to Push a Manual Wheelchair

Consider the attendant's (pusher's) needs when recommending a manual wheelchair (e.g., weight of wheelchair, height of push handle, and ease of folding, lifting, and storage).

Transfers

To transfer independently, the patient must be able to manage all wheelchair parts. Make sure wheelchair components such as wheel locks, seat belts, armrests, and front rigging can be managed independently. Determine what kinds of transfers the patient will be performing so useful features can be ordered for the chair. Regardless of transfer type, wheel locks must be used for safety.

Stand Pivot Transfers

If the patient can stand and pivot during transfers from a wheelchair, make sure armrests are of adequate height and length, wheel locks on both sides of the wheelchair can be reached, casters are in a forward position to reduce the chance of forward tipping[8] (Figure 4-1), and front rigging can swing away (i.e., swing-away footrests) so the patient or assistant does not trip over the footplates (Figure 4-2).

Equipment Considerations

- Height-adjustable full-length armrests
- Swing-away front rigging
- Accessible wheel lock location

---

* Patients included 61 adult wheelchair users with varied diagnoses including postpolio syndrome (PPS), traumatic brain injury (TBI), cerebral vascular accident (CVA), SCI, and cerebral palsy (CP).

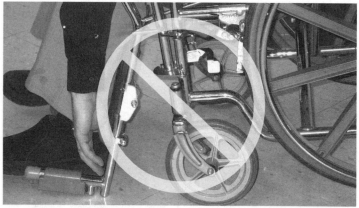

A

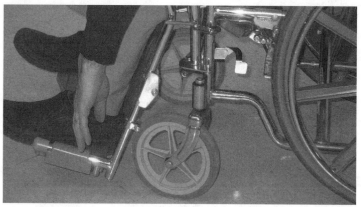

B

FIGURE 4-1 Forward stability and caster position. **(A)** The chair can tip forward when casters are pointing backward. **(B)** When casters are pointing forward, a more stable position is attained for stand pivot transfers.

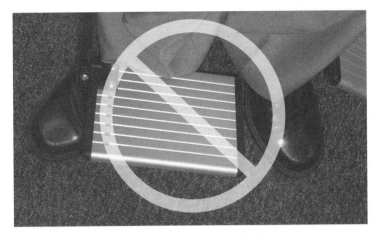

FIGURE 4-2 Avoid tripping over a footrest during stand pivot transfers.

Sliding Board Transfers

If the patient can use a sliding board (i.e., able to slide sideways from a wheelchair to a bed using a shellacked wood board), make sure armrests are removable so the sliding board can be placed under the patient's buttocks. The height difference between the wheelchair seat level and opposing surface should not be too great. The seat surface should also be stable enough during the transfer; foam cushions are generally more stable than air bladder cushions.

Equipment Considerations

- Removable armrests
- Stable seat insert surface

Forward Transfers

Forward transfers, which are commonly performed by patients with bilateral lower limb amputations, enable the patients to transfer out of the wheelchair by positioning the front of the seat flush with the bed and scooting forward. If the patient has front rigging, make sure he or she can swing it completely away from the front of the wheelchair so the seat can be positioned flush and perpendicular with the bed.

Equipment Considerations

- Swing-away or detachable front rigging

Two-Person Transfers

If the patient depends totally on others to be lifted, make sure armrests are removable so caregivers do not have to lift the patient any higher than necessary over obstacles (i.e., the armrests) during the transfer. Removable headrests and swing-away front rigging will enable caregivers to exercise better body mechanics by getting closer to the patient (i.e., closer to the load).

Equipment Considerations

- Removable armrests
- Swing-away front rigging
- Removable headrests

Mechanical Lift Transfers

If the patient is too difficult or too heavy to transfer safely with manual help, consider a mechanical lift. Check the weight capacity of the mechanical lift. Confirm that the patient has sufficient space at home to store and use the lift. Make sure the base of the lift can fit around the wheelchair so the patient can be moved directly over the seat and then properly lowered into the wheelchair. Also ensure everyone is trained to use the lift because tipping and injuries can occur if the lift is not properly used or maintained. Importantly, the patient must be properly positioned in the lift's sling.[8]

Equipment Considerations

- Weight capacity of the lift
- Proper training of caregiver
- Sufficient room in the home for the lift

Car Transfers

If patients lift their wheelchair into a car, consider the following features to make the lift more manageable.[1]

Equipment Considerations

- Folding frame
- Lightweight frame
- Handle on wheelchair—to pull and lift wheelchair into car
- Quick release wheels (see Figure 7-22)
- Removable armrests
- Swing-away, detachable front rigging
- Removable postural inserts

Sitting

How Much Support Is Needed to Sit?

Activity level and trunk control will determine how much back support is needed[9] (Figure 4-3).

Low Back Support

If the patient is very active (in sports) and needs minimal support to sit, a *low back height* will be least restrictive and permit trunk bending, extension, and turning. A back support that is too low, however, may result in back pain.

Midback Support

If the patient self-propels but needs additional trunk support (usually the case), consider a *midback height* (just below the scapula) so that arm, scapula, and upper trunk movements are unrestricted during wheelchair propulsion.

High Back Support

If the patient has poor trunk control and does not self-propel, consider a *high back height* (to acromial level).

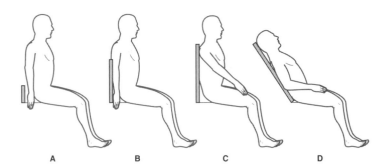

FIGURE 4-3 Back height is determined by amount of trunk control and activity level. **(A)** Low back support provides minimal support for very active patients with good trunk control. **(B)** Midback support provides postural support for the trunk while still allowing unrestricted use of upper extremities during self-propulsion. **(C)** High back support provides maximal postural support for the trunk but may interfere with UE self-propulsion. **(D)** Patients using reclining or tilt wheelchairs need full head and trunk support.

High Back Support and Head Support

Finally, if the patient has poor head control or either reclines or tilts the chair backward in space, a *higher back with a headrest* will be necessary.

Back Height[9]

- *Manual wheelchair users (self-propulsion)*—To inferior angle of scapula or lower
- *Poor trunk control*—To shoulder height
- *Poor head and trunk control*—High back and head support

Determine Head Position for a Comfortable Gaze While Sitting

Normally, with the head vertical, the eyes can gaze comfortably down at objects up to 30 degrees below the horizon.[10]

Upper Limb Function

Manual handrim wheelchair users generally need good UE function.

Can the Patient Use Upper Limbs to Self-Propel?

If the patient self-propels, determine if the patient can reach toward and grasp the handrims, start, stop, and maneuver the wheelchair forward, backwards, on turns, through doorways, up ramps, onto elevators, and later outdoors. Popping wheelies (i.e., balancing the wheelchair only on the rear wheels) is an advanced but necessary wheelchair skill for independence—it is used for quick turning and curb negotiation.

If Self-Propulsion Is Possible, Are Rear Wheels Optimally Positioned?

If the patient can self-propel, make sure the rear wheel axle is ideally positioned relative to the patient's shoulder joint. Otherwise, wheelchair propulsion efficiency may suffer. Unfortunately, the rear wheel axis on a standard (depot) wheelchair is typically aligned with the backpost[11] so the shoulder joint position ends up 2 inches in front of the wheel axis[12]—a distinct disadvantage for propulsion (Figure 4-4).

Altering the position of the rear wheels relative to the seat can affect the energy requirements to self-propel, the maneuverability and stability of the wheelchair, and the weight distribution of the patient in the wheelchair. *Specifically, moving the wheels forward can lead to improved propulsion efficiency, lower rolling resistance, less downhill turning tendency, and improved maneuverability.* Ultralight wheelchairs (see Chapter 6) have this adjustable wheel axle capability but are costly and therefore hard to fund. Brubaker has argued that because of the enhanced wheelchair performance associated with chairs that permit adjustable wheel axle position, we should be required to justify generic wheelchair prescriptions (that don't have this feature) to funding agencies, rather than ultralight/sport chairs (that do).[13]

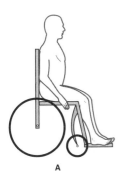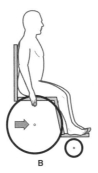

A **B**

FIGURE 4-4 (A) In the standard wheelchair, the rear wheel axis is aligned with the backpost, pushing the patient's shoulder axis 2 inches in front of the wheel axis. Wheelchair propulsion ability may suffer. **(B)** Wheelchair propulsion and maneuverability may improve by adjusting the rear wheel position forward, relative to the patient's seat position in a standard frame.

Research on the optimal wheel position has been investigated most in the paraplegic population.[14] Although wheel axis location should be determined with patient feedback, general guidelines in the literature have included having the rear wheels moved as far anteriorly as the patient can feel comfortable with.[14] (Also see Chapter 7.) Other recommendations include having the shoulder axis placed about 2 inches behind the wheel axis[12] or moving the wheel axis in line with the shoulder, or slightly forward, and adjusting the shoulder–wheel distance such that the elbow is in 30 degrees of flexion when the top of the handrim is grasped.[15]

In summary, to improve self-propulsion ability, consider ordering a wheelchair with adjustable axle hardware. An active user with good trunk balance may benefit by moving the rear wheels/axis forward, although the trade-off will be increased backward chair instability.[16] One solution to this is adding antitippers.

Moving Rear Wheel Axis Forward[11]

- Rolls easier because weight is shifted over the rear wheel axis[16]
- Maneuverability improves if seat position is moved posteriorly relative to wheel axis (reduces moment of inertia)[12]
- Propulsion efficiency improves (i.e., recovery phase of propulsion cycle) if seat position is moved posteriorly relative to wheel axis[12]
- Easier to "pop a wheelie" for curb climbing if seat position is moved posterior relative to wheel axis[12]
- Reduces wheelchair's downhill turning tendency when on sloped surfaces if seat position is moved posteriorly relative to wheel axis[12]
- Shortens the wheel base
- Shorter turning radius
- Reduces stability[12] (easier to tip backward); consider rear antitippers for patient safety

Moving Rear Wheel Axis Backward[16]

- Increases backward stability
- Increases energy required to propel wheelchair
- Increases turning radius

Moving Rear Wheel Axis Upward (or Lowering Seat)[11]

- Stronger stroke propulsion
- Increased trunk stability
- Increased buttocks pressure (due to seat tilt)

What Is the UE Pattern of Propulsion?

Handrim propulsion has two phases: propulsive and recovery. Four propulsion patterns have been identified based on the performance of 38 seasoned SCI manual wheelchair users (11 female; 27 male) with paraplegia ranging in age from 21 to 65 years.[17] The four patterns are: (1) Single looping over propulsion (SLOP): involves hand lifting above the pushrim after the rim release (hand trajectory—a sideways-oriented chocolate kiss candy); (2) Double looping over propulsion (DLOP): involves first lifting the hand above the handrim and then dropping it below during the recovery phase (hand trajectory—a sideways figure eight); (3) Semicircular: involves the hand dropping below the pushrim after rim release (the hand trajectory—an oval or circular pattern); (4) Arcing: the hand pattern follows the shape of the pushrim after rim release (hand trajectory—resembles an arc). Of the four patterns, the *semicircular pattern* was associated with a slower and thus a more desirable push frequency (or cadence) in this SCI population.

Recommendations to Improve SCI Wheelchair Propulsion

Largely based on kinetic and kinematic data involving wheelchair users with paraplegia, the following general recommendations from various authors have been made in order to improve propulsion efficiency and, theoretically, minimize UE injuries associated with manual propulsion:[17–22]

- Apply lower peak forces.
- Slow cadence (push frequency).
- Increase push angle and the time on pushrims, in order to reduce cadence.
- Perform circular propulsive strokes (semicircular pattern) so the hand drops below the pushrim after handrim release.
- Minimize downward directed propulsion forces toward the wheel axle (i.e., "pushing down into the rim").
- Use very light chairs in order to reduce rolling resistance and required propulsion forces.

- Optimize the rear axle placement both vertically and horizontally.
- Lose body weight in order to reduce required propulsion forces.
- Explore pushrim-activated power assist and power wheelchair options.

Hand Grasp and Release Patterns

Evaluating grasp and release patterns on the handrim may also offer insights into propulsion efficiency. In an observational study of pushrim dynamics, 14 persons with MS (8 women, 6 men; ages 48.4 ± 6.3 years; wheelchair use 8.1 ± 9.6 years; severity not reported) demonstrated a nonproductive, "braking effect" during the grasp and release of the pushrims.[23] Wheelchair speeds for this MS group were significantly reduced when compared to an SCI (paraplegia) and a nonneurologically involved group. The MS group also showed fatigue, as evidenced by reduced speed over a 5-minute period while propelling at self-selected speed.

Does the Patient Have Limited Reach?

Limited reach[24,25] can affect a patient's ability to greet people, open doors, push elevator buttons, and retrieve objects from the floor. Wheelchair components such as lap boards, chest harnesses, and seat belts may further restrict the patient's reach ability. Evaluate forward, sideways, backward, and upward upper extremity reach abilities in your patient while he or she remains properly seated in the wheelchair. First, however, ensure the wheelchair is stable in the forward (i.e., point casters forward),[8] sideways, and backward (use rear antitippers) directions. (Wheelchair user manuals may warn against performing some reach maneuvers [e.g., reaching down between knees] that can destabilize the chair.)

ADA recommended limits on reach range for facility access:

- *High forward reach*—48 inches from floor required to reach elevator buttons[25]
- *High side reach*—Up to 54 inches above floor[25]
- *Low forward reach*—No less than 15 inches above floor recommended[25]
- *Low side reach*—No less than 9 inches above floor recommended[25]

- *Backward reach*—Toward utility bag hanging off the back of the wheelchair

Sitting Posture and Reaching

Sitting posture may influence reaching ability in wheelchair users. Sprigle et al. found that pelvic position predicted reaching ability in 20 SCI wheelchair users with tetra- and paraplegia.[26] Posterior pelvic positioning, which was associated with greater reach in this study, may have provided a stable base upon which upper trunk and UEs were able to better function in this population. The downside of posterior pelvic positioning, of course, is an increased risk for pressure ulcer development.

EXERCISES

1. How would you determine whether a manual, power, or attendant-operated wheelchair would be most appropriate for your patient?
2. How would moving the rear wheels forward relative to the seat affect the performance of the wheelchair and the energy requirements of your patient? How would wheelchair stability be affected?
3. What type of armrest and front rigging would you prescribe for patients performing a (a) stand-pivot transfer? (b) sliding board transfer?
4. What two factors should you consider to determine back height for your patient?
5. Sit properly in a stable wheelchair and observe how high and low you reach to the side and forward for objects on the wall (e.g., light switches), on the floor (e.g., boots), or directly in front of you (e.g., a door). Compare your maximal reaching ability with the recommended values for adults reaching while in a standard wheelchair. (Do not reach down between your knees to the floor.)
6. How high must your patient reach to operate the buttons in an elevator?
7. Sit at a desk with your head and trunk vertical (i.e., not leaning forward), hold a book so that you can comfortably read it, and then notice the angle of your eye gaze relative to the horizon. Note how your eyes strain if you move them to look either directly straight ahead or too far down (i.e., below 30 degrees from the horizon)

References

1. Behrman AL. Clinical perspectives on wheelchair selection: factors in functional assessment. *J Rehabil Res Dev.* 1990;2(Supp):17–27.
2. Kilkens OJE, Post MWM, Dallmeijer AJ, Seelen HAM, van der Woude LHV. Wheelchair skills tests: a systematic review. *Clin Rehabil.* 2003;17:418–430.
3. Newton AM, Kirby RL, MacPhee AH, Dupuis DJ, MacLeod DA. Evaluation of manual wheelchair skills: is objective testing necessary or would subjective estimates suffice? *Arch Phys Med Rehabil.* 2002;83:1295–1299.
4. Miles-Tapping C, MacDonald LJ. Lifestyle implications of power mobility. *Phys Occup Ther Geriatr.* 1994;12:31–49.
5. Lange ML. Funding power. *Rehab Manag.* 2005;18(6):34, 36–37.
6. Furumasu J, Guerette P, Tefft D. Relevance of the pediatric powered wheelchair screening test for children with cerebral palsy. *Devel Med Child Neurol.* 2004;46:468–474.
7. Massengale S, Folden D, McConnell P, Stratton L, Whitehead V. Effect of visual perception, visual function, cognition, and personality on power wheelchair use in adults. *Assist Technol.* 2005;17(2):108–121.
8. Batavia M. *Contraindications in Physical Rehabilitation: Doing No Harm.* St. Louis, MO: Saunders; 2006.
9. Kamenetz HL. *The Wheelchair Book: Mobility for the Disabled.* Springfield, CT: CC Thomas; 1969:132–134.

10. Pheasant S. *Body Space: Anthropometry, Ergonomics, and Design.* London: Taylor & Francis; 1996:64.

11. Ragnarsson KT. Clinical perspectives on wheelchair selection: prescription considerations and a comparison of conventional and light weight wheelchairs. *J Rehabil Res Dev.* 1990;2(Supp):8–16.

12. Brubaker C. Ergonometric considerations. *J Rehabil Res Dev.* 1990;2 (Supp):37–48.

13. Brubaker CE. Wheelchair prescription: an analysis of factors that affect mobility and performance. *J Rehab Res Dev.* 1986;23(4):19–26.

14. Boninger ML, Koontz AM, Sisto SA, et al. Pushrim biomechanics and injury prevention in spinal cord injury: recommendations based on CULP-SCI investigations. *J Rehabil Res Dev.* 2005;42(3 Supp 1):9–19.

15. Bergen AF, Presperin J, Tallman T. *Positioning for Function: Wheelchairs and Other Assistive Technologies.* Valhalla, NY: Valhalla Rehabilitation; 1990:77.

16. Currie DM, Hardwick K, Marburger RA, Britell CW. Wheelchair prescription and adaptive seating. In Delisa JL, Gans BM, eds. *Rehabilitation Medicine: Principles and Practice.* 2nd ed. Philadelphia: J B Lippincott; 1993:563–585.

17. Boninger ML, Souza AL, Cooper RA, Fitzgerald SG, Koontz AM, Fay BT. Propulsion patterns and pushrim biomechanics in manual wheelchair propulsion. *Arch Phys Med Rehabil.* 2002;83(5):718–723.

18. Curtis KA, Drysdale GA, Lanza RD, Kolber M, Vitolo RS, West R. Shoulder pain in wheelchair users with tetraplegia and paraplegia. *Arch Phys Med Rehabil.* 1999;80(4):453–457.

19. Ambrosio F, Boninger ML, Souza AL, Fitzgerald SG, Koontz AM, Cooper RA. Biomechanics and strength of manual wheelchair users. *J Spinal Cord Med.* 2005;28(5):407–414.

20. Mercer JL, Boninger M, Koontz A, Ren D, Dyson-Hudson T, Cooper R. Shoulder joint kinetics and pathology in manual wheelchair users. *Clin Biomech.* 2006;21(8):781–789.

21. Boninger ML, Cooper RA, Baldwin MA, Shimada SD, Koontz A. Wheelchair pushrim kinetics: body weight and median nerve function. *Arch Phys Med Rehabil.* 1999;80(8):910–915.

22. Boninger ML, Dicianno BE, Cooper RA, Towers JD, Koontz AM, Souza AL. Shoulder magnetic resonance imaging abnormalities, wheelchair propulsion, and gender. *Arch Phys Med Rehabil.* 2003;84(11):1615–1620. Erratum in: *Arch Phys Med Rehabil.* 2004;85(1):172.

23. Fay BT, Boninger ML, Fitzgerald SG, Souza AL, Cooper RA, Koontz AM. Manual wheelchair pushrim dynamics in people with multiple sclerosis. *Arch Phys Med Rehabil.* 2004;85(6):935–942.

24. Olson SC, Meredith DK. *Wheelchair Interiors.* Chicago: National Easter Seal Society; 1973:5–12.

25. American National Standards Institute. *American National Standard for Buildings and Facilities: Providing Accessibility and Usability for Physically Handicapped People. Accessible Elements and Spaces (A117.1).* New York: American National Standards Institute; 1986:16–73.

26. Sprigle S, Wootten M, Sawacha Z, Thielman G. Relationships among cushion type, backrest height, seated posture, and reach of wheelchair users with spinal cord injury. *J Spinal Cord Med.* 2003;26(3):236–243.

PART III

The Wheelchair

C H A P T E R   5

The Wheelchair: An Introduction

The wheelchair consists of a mobility base and a seating system (Figure 5-1). The *mobility base* (i.e., metal frame) provides the structure and mobility of the wheelchair. Mobility bases will be reviewed in Chapter 6. The *seating system* is mounted into the mobility base and provides postural support for the patient. The seating system and other wheelchair components will be reviewed in Chapter 7.

Indications, contraindications, and risks involved in using wheelchairs and seating systems will be covered in this chapter, along with consideration of wheelchair size, weight, strength, and portability when prescribing. The chapter concludes with a discussion on using ANSI (American National Standards Institute)/RESNA (Rehabilitation Engineering and Assistive Technology Society of North America) wheelchair standards when shopping around for wheelchair features important to the patient.

Indications for a Wheelchair (Mobility Base)

Consider the following indications for a wheelchair that are typically satisfied when a patient can no longer safely and functionally ambulate,[1] even with ambulatory aids. Often, the patient may present with pain, weakness, deformity incoordination, lack of endurance,[2] or loss of a body part.

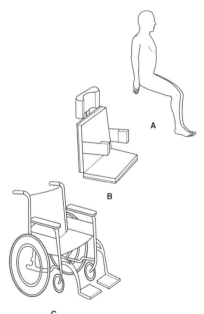

FIGURE 5-1 **(A)** The patient, **(B)** postural support system, and **(C)** mobility base.

- Nonambulatory
- Unsafe/unsteady/nonfunctional ambulator
- Poor cardiopulmonary reserve
- Lower extremity (LE) weight bearing is contraindicated.
- Dependent LE is contraindicated.
- Marginal ambulator—limited to short distances only.

Indications for a Seating System[3]

A seating system may range from the simple to the complex, depending on the patient's needs. At a bare minimum, those who rely on a wheelchair should be provided with an appropriate seat cushion, seat belt, and arm and foot supports.

General Indications

- Improve comfort[4]
- Increase sitting tolerance
- Prevent tissue and pressure damage
- Prevent deformity
- Accommodate or delay progression of an orthopedic deformity[4]
- Decrease pain
- Increase sitting stability
- Enhance respiratory function
- Enhance mobility through positioning
- Enhance functional abilities
- May improve body image
- Minimize influence of abnormal tone and reflexes[4]

Contraindications for Using a Wheelchair[5,6]

- *Any condition where sitting is contraindicated:* Wheelchair use occurs from a sitting position. An ischial pressure ulcer can therefore be considered as an absolute contraindication for wheelchair use, that is, sitting on the ulcer. (In this case, locomoting prone on a gurney may be an option until healing occurs.)
- *Manual propulsion:* For manual wheelchair propulsion, poor judgment and blindness are additional absolute contraindications. Other relative contraindications may include vertebral fractures, orthopedic postoperative conditions, disc nerve compression, trunk weakness, and postural defects. (The latter two concerns may merely suggest the need for appropriate postural support.)
- *Power mobility:* For power chair or scooter use, in addition to ischial pressure ulcers, poor judgment and blindness, inattention, irresponsibility, and an inability to voluntarily control and operate power switches are contraindications.

Risks of Wheelchair Use[1]

The benefits of wheeled mobility need to be weighed against the risks described below.

- *Deaths:* Wheelchair-related deaths are well documented; 770 wheelchair–related fatalities occurred in the United States between 1973 and 1987, based on death certificates. Most (77%) were associated with tips and falls. Some of the remaining causes included stair injuries, burns, and restraint-related asphyxia.[7] The Food and Drug Administration reported approximately 18 manual wheelchair–related deaths, 23 power wheelchair–related deaths, and 30 scooter–related deaths from September 1986 to November 2002, April 1990 to March 2003, and November 1986 to January 2003, respectively.[5]

- *Acute injuries:* The number of wheelchair-related U.S. emergency room visits doubled to 100,000 visits over the past decade, according to a study using 2003 data from the National Electronic Injury Surveillance System (NEISS). Xiang et al. reported 65% to 80% of the injuries were tip and fall-related.[8] For children, ages 6 to 17 years (mostly boys), the injuries tended to occur more outdoors in association with ramps, curbs, and stairs. For adults and children under 6 years of age, the injuries occurred more at home or within institutions.

- *Repetitive UE injuries:* Manual wheelchair use has been linked to repetitive injury–related pathologies of the UE (i.e., repetitive strain injuries).[9] The problem is well documented in the spinal cord injury (SCI) population and may in part be related to handrim propulsion, which by nature is a very repetitive activity. For example, Curtis et al. found 78% of the tetraplegic and 59% of the paraplegic sample reported shoulder pain since receiving their wheelchair.[10]

  Push rim forces have been linked to pathological changes in the UE of persons with paraplegia. Mercer et al. found that the level of joint forces occurring in the shoulder during handrim propulsion were associated with the presence of MRI-detected shoulder pathology (i.e., edema, thickening) in 33 persons with paraplegia.[11] Boninger et al. found that rapid loading of the pushrims during propulsion was associated with median nerve function in 34 persons with paraplegia, suggesting a possible higher risk of developing median nerve injuries in this group.[12]

- *Pressure ulcers:* In the United States, pressure ulcer incidence has been reported as high as 23.9% and 38% in long-term and acute care facilities, respectively, despite being relatively stable over the past decade or so.[13] Many wheelchair users are at high risk for developing pressure ulcers (see Chapter 3) because of associated motor and sensory impairment.

- *Latex-related allergies:* Latex can be found in wheelchair tires and positional devices (cushions, seat backs) and may result in skin rashes, and respiratory symptoms. In extreme cases, latex exposure can lead to anaphylactic shock, although this may be more of a concern with surgically implanted prosthetics.[14] Children with spina bifida are particularly susceptible.[14]

- *Electromagnetic interference (EMI):* Power wheelchairs and scooters may be susceptible to EMI from environmental sources such as power lines or even household electronic products. Interference with the operation of control circuitry can lead to erratic wheelchair behavior.[15]
- *Disuse atrophy and deconditioning:* Passive wheelchair users can lead a sedentary lifestyle. For all its efficiency shortcomings, handrim manual propulsion still provides a benefit of exercise, whereas power mobility does not.
- *Hip and knee flexion contractures:* Long-term wheelchair positioning places hip and knee flexors in a chronically shortened posture. Alternative positioning such as supported standing programs and standing wheelchairs may help counter the ill effects of prolonged sitting.
- *Dependency on wheelchair:* Some patients may become overly reliant on their wheelchairs.

Dimension, Weight, Strength, Transportation, and Appearance

Critical factors to consider before prescribing any wheelchair follow.

Wheelchair Size

The size of the wheelchair is determined, of course, by the size of the patient (see Chapter 3). Record the patient's seat width, seat depth, back height, and heel-to-knee measurement.[16,17] Be aware that frame size names and dimensions may vary among manufacturers. This list, however, should give you a starting point when communicating with suppliers.

- *Preschool size*—10" seat width and 8" seat depth[16]
- *Pediatric size*—12" to 14" seat width and 11½" seat depth[17]
- *Junior size*—16" seat width and 14" seat depth[16]
- *Narrow adult size*—16" seat width and 16" seat depth[17]
- *Adult size*—18" seat width and 16" seat depth[16]
- *Tall adult size*—18" seat width and 17" seat depth[17]
- *Wide adult size*—20" to 28" seat width and 16" seat depth[1,16]

Wheelchair Width

In general, do not make the wheelchair any wider than absolutely necessary because it can affect accessibility and propulsion ability (wheels further away from UEs). A standard wheelchair outside width is 26 inches.[18] Widening the chair substantially may result in an inability to clear front doorways of a home or fit onto the ramp dimension of some ambulettes. (I had personal experience with the latter.)

Narrowing devices, which use a gear/crank mechanism, have been used on frames to temporarily narrow the wheelchair width a few inches for clearance.[16] If the wheelchair is too narrow, however, the frame may be too unstable and the patient could tip over sideways. If this is the case, consider moving the wheels out to the side, angling the rear wheels (camber), or getting a wider frame to improve stability—but do so with much thought (i.e., measure all relevant environments).

Wide Wheelchair Problems

- Difficulty reaching handrims to self-propel
- Hard to clear doorways
- Hard to fit on narrow ambulette ramps
- Less postural stability and increased risk of scoliosis if no postural supports on wheelchair[1]

Wheelchair Height

The standard seat height is 19 inches from the floor. A cushion will probably raise the seat height further. Taller patients often need a higher seat position. If the wheelchair seat is too high, however, it may be difficult for caregivers to see where they are going when pushing the wheelchair from behind. These wheelchairs may also require a higher van roof for head clearance. Also, push propulsion mechanics may suffer because the UEs are moved further away from the handrims.[19] A higher seat may also be less stable for the patient. Finally, be aware of the effect of seat height on table height level, knee clearance under tables, transfer height from floor, and social intercourse (eye level).

High Wheelchair Seat Problems

- Higher center of gravity and less stability.
- Difficult for short caregivers to see ahead while pushing wheelchair.
- Head level may be too high for clearance on low roof vans.
- Difficulty reaching floor for foot-assisted propulsion.
- Table height may be too low for patients.
- Knee level may be too high for clearance under a table.
- Transfers may be more difficult for short patients.
- Pushrim biomechanics may suffer.

Children and shorter adults often need a lower seat height. If the wheelchair/ seat is too low, tall caregivers may strain to push the wheelchair. This is also true if the wheelchair frame tilts backward, which lowers the push handle's position toward the floor. Stroller handle attachments can be ordered to raise the position of the push handles.

Low Wheelchair Seat Problems

- Tall caregivers may strain to push the wheelchair.
- Front rigging may drag on ground if lowered to accommodate patient's leg length.
- Table level may be too high.
- Transfers may be difficult for tall patients.

How High Should the Push Handles Be?

The push handle height of a standard adult wheelchair is 3 feet from the floor. To determine optimal push handle height for a particular caregiver, calculate 70% to 80% of the caregiver's floor to shoulder height.[20] For example, if the floor to shoulder height of a caregiver measures 40 inches, then the push handle height would be about 70% of 40 inches, or 28 inches from the floor (40 × (0.70) = 28 inches). Determine if this calculated height is a comfortable push handle height for the caregiver and if the supplier can order push handles close to that height. Alternatively, you can simply ask the caregiver what push handle height would be comfortable for pushing the wheelchair.

Wheelchair Weight

The rule is, the more components you have, the heavier the wheelchair will be. A heavier wheelchair often means more effort for starts and stops and greater rolling resistance. You can gain an appreciation of wheelchair weight by pushing one around all day—it's a lot of work. Don't take away the patient's propulsion function by making the wheelchair too heavy.

Strength/Construction

The strength required for the frame depends on the user's activity level, body weight, and terrain. Heavy duty frames should be considered for patients who are heavy (heavy duty frames come in increasing levels of weight capacity), exhibit very strong extensor activity, or propel under rugged terrain conditions. Frames with higher weight capacities may have reinforced joints, double cross-braces, and steel construction. Ultralight frames, on the other hand, may be durable *and* light but with limited weight capacity.[21] The durability of a frame depends not only on the type of materials used (e.g., titanium, steel), but also on how the chairs are designed (e.g., material thickness, cross-sectional area) and put together (e.g., welding/preheating techniques).[22]

Indications for Heavy Duty Construction

- Heavy patients; obese (bariatric) patients
- Strong extensor tone or activity
- Heavy outdoor use
- Rough outdoor terrain

Disadvantages of Heavy Duty Construction

- Increased weight capacity may also mean increased frame width (and potential access problems, e.g., doorways).
- Heavy chairs have great rolling resistance—harder to propel.
- Cost

Portability

Wheelchairs that fold and have removable components are more easily stored during transportation.

Rigid Versus Nonfolding Frames[23]

- Rigid (nonfolding) frames do not fold and are generally more durable and lighter than folding frames but less portable.
- Folding frames can be stored and transported in small spaces. Standard frames fold toward the middle like an accordion or director's chair (Figure 5-2A). The back posts of tilt-in-space frames, on the other hand, fold forward onto themselves like a suitcase (Figure 5-2B).

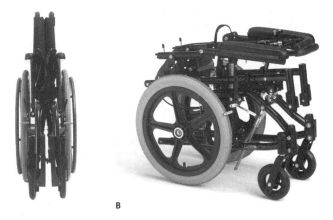

A   B

FIGURE 5-2 (A) Standard frames fold toward the middle like an accordion or director's chair. **(B)** Tilt-in-space frames fold forward onto themselves. (Courtesy of Sunrise Medical)

Detachable Wheelchair Components
Wheelchairs can also be made lighter and more portable during transportation by removing components from the frame.

- Quick release rear wheels (see Figure 7-22)
- Removable seat and back inserts
- Removable head supports
- Detachable front rigging
- Removable armrests

Transportation

School Bus Transportation

In 2008, the American Academy of Pediatrics reaffirmed its 2001 recommendations regarding school bus transportation, including for those with special needs traveling in a wheelchair.[24,25]

> If a child can be reasonably transferred from their wheelchair to a FMVSS213-compliant child restraint system, they should be transferred, facing forward, for transportation.

Otherwise, they should use "certified transit wheelchairs" when traveling on a school bus whenever possible. If the patient is ordering a wheelchair and will be traveling on a bus in a wheelchair, inquire about transit options from the manufacturer that are SAE J2249 crash-tested compliant, approved by ANSI/RESNA standard WC19, and constructed with dedicated tie-down securement locations on the wheelchair frame.[26] Occupied wheelchairs must be secured in a forward position by the frame (not wheels) to the floor of a bus using four approved straps (wheelchair tie-down) .

Occupants should be restrained by a separate device (occupant restraint system), with a shoulder harness (upper torso) and pelvis (lower torso) restraints.

Liquid oxygen tanks, lap boards, and unoccupied wheelchairs should be stored and secured to prevent them from becoming projectiles. Headrests provide needed support for the patient's head during transportation.[26]

Air Travel and Battery Storage

Airlines have regulations for storing wheelchair batteries, which can typically be viewed on their Web sites (e.g., for Southwest Airlines, go to http://www.southwest.com/travel_center/disability.html). Wet cell batteries, for example, may need to be removed from the wheelchair and stored in a "protective battery box" as per federal HAZMAT safety regulations. If a battery is not labeled nonspillable, procedures for dangerous goods packaging also may apply. Nonspillable batteries may not need to be removed from the wheelchair but may still need their battery cables disconnected to prevent potential electrical fires.[27]

Appearance (Ugly as Sin Factor)

The look of a chair may be more important to the patient than the therapist.[28,29] In fact, patients may hate the way a chair looks.[31] As a person with an SCI expressed in a Netherlands questionnaire regarding wheelchair appearance: "You look like an idiot in that thing."[30 (p 113)]

Because client tastes and self-image are factors in wheelchair selection,[32] it is always a good idea to involve the patient in these choices.

Shopping for Wheelchairs: ANSI/RESNA Wheelchair Standards

All wheelchairs do not perform equally. Some chairs are more durable, others quicker, and still others more stable. To help you decide on the tradeoffs among similar models,[31] RESNA in conjunction with the American National Standards Institute (ANSI) has developed voluntary performance and safety standards for wheelchair manufacturers. (International and European standards also exist.) Standards testing is somewhat analogous to crash testing in the automobile industry or product testing from *Consumer Reports*. Tests are standardized by evaluating wheelchair performance under uniform, predetermined conditions [32,33] which result in either a pass/fail outcome (e.g., fabric ignites/does not ignite) or a score with relative meaning (e.g., maximal speed is 8 mph). The outcomes of tested wheelchair models is published in peer-reviewed medical literature, some of which will be reviewed in Chapter 7.[22,34,35]

The wheelchair standards are useful when comparison shopping to determine which wheelchair (within a similar model and price range) performs best for a feature *important to a particular patient's lifestyle.* For a person with a very active lifestyle (8 hours a day, outdoor use), weight and durability may rank high in priorities. But for a patient who lives in a very hilly environment, stability and power (for power chairs) may be more important. In fact, I had a friend who received a low-end power chair that performed well in New York City, but poorly when he moved to San Francisco. The chair could no longer make it up the hills, which were far steeper in the Bay Area. So comparing power performance of different models using the ANSI/RESNA wheelchair standards would have been helpful in my friend's situation.

Problems are encountered when attempting to use ANSI/RESNA wheelchair standards to comparison shop. First, the manufacturer's compliance with the standards is voluntary, and their test results may not be readily available to consumers for a number of reasons, such as losing a competitive edge, attracting insurance scrutiny, and increasing litigation exposure.[22,34,35] Second, existing standards may not be comprehensive enough to keep pace with burgeoning technological advances in the wheelchair industry. Third, the standards may not be stringent enough.[34] Despite these limitations, Medicare is currently applying some standards (e.g., weight capacity, curb climbing) when coding products (HICPIC coding system) for reimbursement/funding.[34]

Some wheelchair standards, as described in the literature, are briefly described in the following sections. For a comprehensive and detailed review of protocols and interpretation, refer to publications such as the *ANSI/RESNA Wheelchair Standards: Sample Evaluation and Guide to Interpreting Test Data for Prescribing Power Wheelchairs*.[36]

Wheelchair Standards: Manual Wheelchairs

Dimensional, performance, and safety questions to consider for manual wheelchairs follow. To evoke a comparative shopping mindset, add the phrase "compared to similar models" when asking the following questions.[32,33]

What Are the Dimensions and Weight of the Wheelchair?

The amount of space required to store the assembled, disassembled, or folded wheelchair while in an airplane, car, or closet may be important to you. By the same token, you may wish to know how heavy the frame and each of its components are for carrying up stairs, lifting into a car, and propelling on level surfaces. In fact, chair weight has important implications for propulsion efficiency because it adds to rolling resistance.[32,33]

Stability: How Stable (or Tippy) Is the Wheelchair in a Forward, Backward, or Sideways Direction?

In other words, how safe is the chair on ramps, hills, and when leaning off to the side. The test involves placing the wheelchair on an adjustable incline surface, facing up, down, or sideways, and determining at what angles the wheels first lift off the surface. Wheelchairs that lift off the surface at milder slopes are considered less stable.[32,33]

How Well Does the Wheelchair Resist Tips and Rolls on a Hill While the Wheel Locks Are Engaged?

This is important if the patient frequents hilly terrain. The test involves placing the wheelchair on a slope with wheel locks engaged and determining at what angle the chair begins to slide/roll/tip. Wheel locks are deemed more effective if slides/rolls/tips occur at steeper slopes.[32,33]

Fatigue Testing: How Durable Is the Wheelchair When Repeatedly Rolling Over a Bumpy Surface (Double Drum Fatigue Test) or When Repeatedly Dropped from a Small Height (Curb Drop Test)?

These tests will provide information about durability. With a 100-kg test dummy in the seat, the wheelchair is placed on two drums with slats to simulate a bumpy, rough ride at a speed of 1 m/s for 200,000 cycles. If the double drum test is successfully completed, the wheelchair is then dropped 6,666 times from a 50-mm height. The double drum and drop test sequence is repeated until damage is observed The chair that completes more cycles without damage is considered more durable.[35,37] From a real-life perspective, 200,000 drum cycles and 6,666 drop tests are equivalent to traveling 100 miles on rough terrain.[22]

Static and Impact Testing: How Well Does the Wheelchair or Component Resist Static and Impact Loads?

This question has relevance for the patient's family who carry the chair up flights of steps (exerting static or hold forces on components) or the patient who has a tendency to crash into obstacles (exerting temporary forces on components). Static strength tests can involve applying a constant force (ranging from 440 N to 1,000 N) to armrests, footrests, and push handles for 5 seconds. Impact strength tests can involve applying a weighted pendulum (e.g., 10 to 25 kg) to components such as backrests, footrests, and casters. Evaluation of strength is based on the presence or absence of any permanent damage to components.[37]

Maneuverability: Using a Three-Point Maneuver, How Well Can the Wheelchair Turn Around in a Hallway?

For the patient who lives in a studio or other small living space, this test may be important. The narrowest corridor width under which the wheelchair can complete the task is reported.[32,33]

Flammability: Is the Manufacturer's Upholstery Flame (Ignition) Resistant?

This is important for patients who smoke, for visitors who smoke in proximity to the wheelchair, and for patients who spend time near a stove. The test involves trying to ignite wheelchair fabric to see if it catches on fire or only smolders.[32,33]

Wheelchair Standards: Power Wheelchairs and Power-Operated Vehicles (POVs)

For power chairs and POVs, performance and safety questions to consider are briefly described in the following sections. Dimensions, weight, flammability, durability, fatigue, static stability, and hallway maneuverability standards have already been described under manual wheelchairs. Other standards include battery and electrical system safety and finger entrapment protection. (The latter is important for households with children.)

Speed: How Quickly Can the Power Chair Advance Forward, Reverse, and Accelerate?

Speed and acceleration may be important for timed outdoor activities such as street crossings. Power chairs will not need to exceed 5 mph indoors but should exceed this speed outdoors.[32,36]

Obstacle Climbing: How High a Step Can the Power Chair Climb?

Curb climbing performance may be important if ramp and curb cuts are commonly unavailable in the patient's neighborhood (e.g., car blocking access). The height of climb is reported.[32,33,36]

Range: How Far Can the Chair Travel on One Battery Charge?

Patients who travel great distances in a single day will find this measure important. The test involves traveling on a test course at maximal speed; total distance is then estimated.

Climatic Test: How Well Does the Chair Operate Under Conditions of Rain or Temperature Extremes?

These tests may be important depending on where you live. The tests can involve exposing the wheelchair to water (for 10 minutes), cold temperatures (around –25° C for at least 3 hours), hot temperatures (around 50° C for at least 3 hours), and heat and cold storage (about –40° C and 65° C for at least 5 hours). Wheelchair function is checked following each exposure.[36,37]

Dynamic Stability: How Stable (Tippy) Is the Power Chair Traveling at Maximal Speed When Braking on Slopes of Various Angles?

The slope angle at which the wheels lift off the floor surface is reported.[36,37]

Effectiveness of Brakes: How Long Does It Take To Stop While Running at Maximal Speed?

This clearly has to do with crash prevention. I knew a person with tetraplegia who shattered a toe (subsequently amputated) because his power chair did not stop until his foot pummeled into the rear wall of the elevator. The test involves engaging the brakes while the chair, with a seated 100-kg test dummy, ascends and descends slopes at varying angles. The distance following braking is recorded.[36,37]

How Much Force Is Necessary to Manually Push the Power Chair?

This is important if the battery dies when outdoors and a caregiver needs to push the chair home. Recorded force levels are compared against a criterion value.[36]

References

1. Kamenetz HL. *The Wheelchair Book: Mobility for the Disabled.* Springfield, CT: CC Thomas; 1969:132–148.
2. Freney D. Pediatric Seating. *Home Health Care Dealer/Supplier.* 1995;Sept/Oct:103–105.
3. Kohlmeyer KM, Yarkony GM. Functional outcomes after spinal cord injury rehabilitation. In Yarkony GM, ed. *Spinal Cord Injury: Medical Management and Rehabilitation.* Gaithersburg, MD: Aspen; 1994; 9–14.
4. Taylor SJ. Evaluating the client with physical disabilities for wheelchair sitting. *Am J Occup Ther.* 1987;41:711–716.
5. Batavia M. *Contraindications in Physical Rehabilitation: Doing No Harm.* St. Louis, MO: Saunders; 2006.
6. Tan JC. *Practical Manual of Physical Medicine and Rehabilitation: Diagnostics, Therapeutics, and Basic Problems.* St. Louis, MO: Mosby; 1998.
7. Calder CJ, Kirby RL. Fatal wheelchair–related accidents in the United States. *Am J Phys Med Rehabil.* 1990;69(4):184–190.
8. Xiang H, Chany A-M, Smith GA. Wheelchair related injuries treated in US emergency departments. *Inj Prev.* 2006;12(1):8–11.
9. Levy CE, Chow JW. Pushrim-activated power-assist wheelchairs: elegance in motion. *Am J Phys Med Rehabil.* 2004;83(2):166–167.
10. Curtis KA, Drysdale GA, Lanza RD, Kolber M, Vitolo RS, West R. Shoulder pain in wheelchair users with tetraplegia and paraplegia. *Arch Phys Med Rehabil.* 1999;80(4):453–457.
11. Mercer JL, Boninger M, Koontz A, Ren D, Dyson-Hudson T, Cooper R. Shoulder joint kinetics and pathology in manual wheelchair users. *Clin Biomech.* 2006;21:781–789.
12. Boninger ML, Cooper RA, Baldwin MA, Shimada SD, Koontz A. Wheelchair pushrim kinetics: body weight and median nerve function. *Arch Phys Med Rehabil.* 1999;80:910–915.
13. Zulkowski K, Langemo D, Posthauer ME, National Pressure Ulcer Advisory Panel. Coming to consensus on deep tissue injury. *Advances Skin Wound Care.* 2005;18(1):28–29.
14. Scoggin AE, Parks KM. Latex sensitivity in children with spina bifida: implications for occupational therapy practitioners. *Am J Occup Ther.* 1997;51(7):608–611.
15. Witters DM, Ruggera PS. Electromagnetic compatibility (EMC) of powered wheelchairs and scooters. Proceedings of the RESNA Annual Conference; June 18–22, 1994;14:359–360.
16. Wilson AB, McFarland SR. Types of wheelchairs. *J Rehabil Res Dev.* 1990:2. Clinical Supplement 104–116.
17. Nassie M, Personal communication, September 8, 1997.
18. American National Standards Institute. *American National Standard for Buildings and Facilities: Providing Accessibility and Usability for Physically Handicapped People. Accessible Elements and Spaces (A117.1).* New York: American National Standards Institute; 1986:16–73.
19. Van der Woude LH, Veeger D-J, Rozendal RH. Seat height in handrim wheelchair propulsion. *J Rehabil Res Devel.* 1989;26(4):31–50.
20. Pheasant S. *Body Space: Anthropometry, Ergonomics, and Design.* London: Taylor & Francis; 1996:132.

21. Medicare Rights Center. Forcing isolation: Medicare's "in the home" coverage standard for wheelchairs. *Care Manage J*. 2005;6(1):29–37.

22. Cooper RA, Robertson RN, Lawrence B, et al. Life cycle analysis of depot versus rehabilitation manual wheelchairs. *J Rehabil Res Dev*. 1996;33(1):45–55.

23. Smith R. A lightweight option. *Rehab Manage*. 2008;21(3):18, 20, 22.

24. American Academy of Pediatrics. Policy statement. February and May 2008. Available at: http://aappolicy.aappublications.org/cgi/content/full/pediatrics;122/2/450. Accessed November 6, 2008.

25. Committee on Injury and Poison Prevention. School bus transportation of children with special health care. *Pediatrics*. 2001;108:516–518.

26. Zimmerman JM. Get on the bus. *Rehab Manage*. 2003;16(7):48–51, 74.

27. Southwest Airlines. Traveling tips for customers with disabilities: manual and power wheelchairs. Available at: http://www.southwest.com/travel_center/disability.html#wheelchairs. Accessed November 4, 2008.

28. Batavia M, Batavia AI, Friedman R. Changing chairs: anticipating problems in prescribing chairs. *Disability Rehabil*. 2001;23(12):539–548.

29. Mortenson WB, Miller WC. The wheelchair procurement process: perspectives of clients and prescribers. *Can J Occup Ther*. 2008;75(3):167–175.

30. Post MW, van Asbeck FW, van Dijk AJ, Schrijvers AJ. Services for spinal cord injured: availability and satisfaction. *Spinal Cord*. 1997;35(2):109–115.

31. Pearlman JL, Cooper RA, Karnawat J, Cooper R, Boninger ML. Evaluation of the safety and durability of low-cost nonprogrammable electric powered wheelchairs. *Arch Phys Med Rehabil*. 2005;86(12):2361–2370.

32. McLaurin CA, Axelson P. Wheelchair standards: an overview. *J Rehabil Res Dev*. 1990;2(Supp):100–103.

33. Axelson P, Minkel J, Chesney D. *A Guide to Wheelchair Selection: How to Use the ANSI/RESNA Wheelchair Standards to Buy a Wheelchair*. Washington, DC: Paralyzed Veterans of America; 1994.

34. Cooper RA. Wheelchair standards: it's all about quality assurance and evidence-based practice. *J Spinal Cord Med*. 2006;29(2):93–94.

35. Cooper RA, Gonzalez J, Lawrence B, Renschler A, Boninger ML, VanSickle DP. Performance of selected lightweight wheelchairs on ANSI/RESNA tests. *Arch Phys Med Rehabil*. 1997;78:1138–1144.

36. The ANSI/RESNA wheelchair standards: sample evaluation and guide to interpreting test data for prescribing power wheelchairs. *Health Devices*. 1993;22(10):432–484.

37. Rentschler AJ, Cooper RA, Fitzgerald SG, et al. Evaluation of selected electric-powered wheelchairs using the ANSI/RESNA standards. *Arch Phys Med Rehabil*. 2004;85(4):611–619.

CHAPTER 6

The Mobility Base

A mobility base is the structural foundation of the wheelchair (the metal frame) that provides locomotion for the patient. Mobility bases typically also include armrests, casters, rear wheels, handrims, front rigging, wheel locks, and a sling-upholstered seat and back.

Mobility base decisions are determined primarily by (1) how the patient will propel the chair (e.g., manually, powered, attendant-assisted) and (2) body orientation needs (e.g., tilt, recline, elevation, standing). Another important set of factors are performance (e.g., durability, power), safety (e.g., stability), and chair dimensions (e.g., frame size, mass, weight capacity). Review American National Standards Institute/Rehabilitation and Assistive Technology Center of North America (ANSI/RESNA) wheelchair standards when comparison shopping. Finally, consider product availability, warranty, and dealer support.[1]

Mobility Bases That Address Different Manual Propulsion Needs

Standard Frame (Institutional, Depot)

Standard or conventional frames are your basic nonadjustable wheelchair—the kind you might view through the drugstore window or see in institutions and hospitals (also called depot-style wheelchairs) (Figure 6-1A).

Although low in initial purchase cost, institutional depot-type wheelchairs can be substantially less durable and result ultimately in higher life cycle costs (costly upkeep) for long-time users. Cooper et al. subjected six steel depot wheelchairs (38-lb weight) to ANSI/RESNA standard fatigue testing.[2] All six sustained class 3 permanent damage including some frame failures.

Because depot chairs are relatively heavy, not very adjustable (i.e., fixed axle position), and have high life cycle costs (not very durable) they are not a good choice for an active or long-term wheelchair user.

Typical Dimensions

A standard adult wheelchair has an outside width of a little more than 2 feet and a 4-foot length. Push handles are 3 feet from the floor and the seat is a little more than 1½ feet from the floor.[3,4]

- Outside width in rear = 26 inches
- Outside width in front = 18 inches
- Length of wheelchair = 48 inches
- Push handles = 36 inches from the floor
- Armrests = 30 inches from the floor
- Seat = 19 inches from the floor

Requirements

- 90 degrees of hip flexion
- 70-degree popliteal angles (i.e., adequate hamstring length). If knee flexion contractures are present, 90-degree front rigging may be required to support the feet.
- Good head control

Hemiplegic Chairs (Footdrive)

Hemiplegic chairs are ordered if the patient needs a frame low enough to the floor to reach the ground for foot propulsion. The seat is 2 inches lower than a standard frame seat, the tires are smaller (i.e., 22-inch diameter rather than 24-inch),[3] and the front rigging is specially adapted.[3]

Stroke patients frequently use this frame. The hemiplegic frame is also useful for the shorter patient who needs a low seat level for transfers. If the patient needs to be close to the floor, this wheelchair may be appropriate (Figure 6-1B).

Indications

- Foot propulsion
- Hemiplegic patients
- Transfers for short patients

Disadvantages

- Taller individuals may have difficulty standing during transfers due to the lower seat level.
- Tables may be too high while sitting in this wheelchair.

Lightweight Wheelchairs

Lightweight wheelchairs generally weigh less than the standard/institutional/depot-type chairs and may offer some limited adjustability (e.g., offering several rear axle positions on some models) (Figure 6-2).

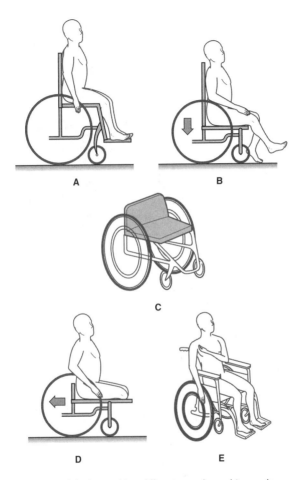

FIGURE 6-1 Some mobility bases address different manual propulsion needs. **(A)** The standard wheelchair frame requires the patient to have at least 90-degree hip flexion. **(B)** The hemiplegic chair is lower to the ground to enable foot propulsion. **(C)** Ultralight frames provide maneuverability and speed for the very active patient with low postural needs. **(D)** The amputee frame moves the rear wheels posteriorly to improve backward stability and to reduce the possibility of tipping the wheelchair backward. (E) The one-hand-drive wheelchair allows the patient with hemiplegia to self-propel a wheelchair using two handrims located on the same wheel.

FIGURE 6-2 High-strength lightweight wheelchair. (Courtesy of Sunrise Medical)

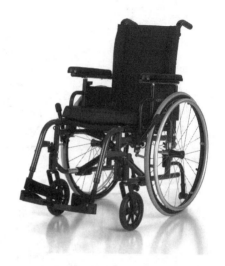

Lightweight wheelchairs may have a speed advantage over heavier chairs. Parziale found that the time to travel 400 feet (at a sprint pace) on an indoor lino-leum floor was shorter in a spinal cord injury (SCI) population using a lightweight wheelchair as compared with a standard wheelchair.[5] Although the effect was noted in all groups (i.e., tetraplegia, high paraplegia [T1–6], and low paraplegia [T7–L4]; $n = 26$; $P \leq 0.01$) it was largest for the tetraplegia group (standard 72.3 ± 20.8 seconds vs. lightweight 55.7 ± 3.9 seconds). The majority of participants in a posttest questionnaire also preferred the lightweight over the standard wheelchair, although respondents were not blinded to chair type.

Although selected lightweight wheelchairs perform similarly during fatigue testing, they are not exceptionally durable. Cooper et al. found only 1 of 9 chairs from various manufacturers passed all ANSI/RESNA fatigue tests and that more than half of the chairs sustained frame failure.[1]

Ultralight Frames (Sports Chairs)

Ultralight frames are the "holy grail" among many long-term highly active manual wheelchair users because of their very lightweight characteristics (<30 lbs without armrests and foot supports),[6] generous adjustability, ease in maneuverability, and speed. As a result, they are very popular for sports and among the paraplegic population (Figures 6-1C and 6-3). Obtaining funding for ultralight wheelchairs, however, is difficult due to their higher costs.

Although they weigh less than a standard frame, ultralights are not for every-one because the frame may have a limited weight capacity. In addition, they may not offer sufficient postural support. Adding supports would, of course, result in a heavier frame.

Energy Efficiency and Ultralights

Ultralight wheelchair propulsion may be more energy efficient than standard wheelchairs for the SCI population. Beekman et al. reported that SCI persons who propelled over 20 minutes did so with higher self-selected speeds and greater outdoor distances using a 27-lb ultralight wheelchair compared with a 44-lb standard wheelchair.[7] The participants (44 paraplegia, 30 tetraplegia, C6 or lower) were mostly males who recently finished in-patient rehabilitation, had complete (motor injuries), and ranged in age from 17–50 years. For tetraplegia, mean distance and speed were standard 891.9 ± 216.2 meters vs. ultralight 958.7 ± 256.8 meters and standard 45.8 ± 11.1 m/s vs. ultralight 49.0 ± 213.4 m/s, respectively. For paraplegia, mean distance and speed were standard 1,379.4 ± 249.0 meters vs. ultralight 1,534.9 ± 275.55 meters and standard 69.9 ± 12.5 m/s vs. ultralight 79.2 ± 14.3 m/s, respectively. Importantly, the group with paraplegia also showed lower mean oxygen costs using the ultralight when compared with using the standard chair (standard 0.16 ± 0.02 ml/kg/m vs. ultralight 0.13 ± 0.02 ml/kg/m).

Life Cycle Costs, Value, and Ultralights

Ultralight wheelchairs are relatively durable but do vary in quality. Using ANSI/RESNA standards, Cooper et al. found that four ultralight wheelchair models (*n* = 12) from different manufacturers were significantly different on fatigue tests and life cycle costs (1999 data).[8] Nevertheless, although the initial purchase of

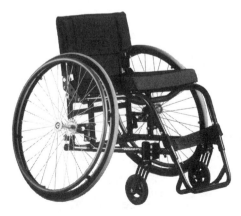

FIGURE 6-3 Ultralight wheelchair. (Courtesy of Sunrise Medical)

ultralight wheelchairs is expensive, they are more durable and have a longer fatigue life when compared with lightweight and depot-type wheelchairs.

Comparative outcomes on fatigue testing across studies have revealed that ultralight chairs have a longer fatigue life (894,500 total cycles) than lightweight chairs (187,370 total cycles), which in turn have a longer fatigue life than depot-institutional type wheelchairs (56,139 total cycles).[1] Thus, ultralight wheelchairs may be the best value of the three categories for long-term users. Because these chairs are highly adjustable, ultralight wheelchairs can be configured to minimize rolling resistance (making it easier to propel) and therefore may require less harmful pushrim forces that are associated with UE repetitive injuries in manual wheelchair users.

Indications

- Very active, long-term wheelchair users
- Energy-efficient propulsion (lightweight)
- Activities requiring speed or quick maneuverability

Advantages

- Lightweight materials—aluminum alloy, titanium, graphite[4]
- Strong frame
- Multiple adjustable axle positions,[4] to improve propulsion performance

Disadvantages

- Cost
- Decreased postural and foot support
- Limited weight capacity
- Storage problem (if unable to fold rigid frame)
- Rough ride (if rigid frame)

Racing Wheelchair Characteristics[4]

- Rear wheels = 26–27 inches
- Narrow, high pressure tires (160 psi)
- Small handrims = 12 inches
- Large casters with precision bearing—improve rolling performance
- Low seat—top of wheel is located near the axilla; improved stability

Amputee Frame (or Amputee Axle Kits)

The amputee frame or amputee axle conversion kit positions the rear wheels at least 1 inch posteriorly to shift the chair's center of gravity, improve the stability, and reduce the chance of the wheelchair tipping backward.[3] This frame may be considered if the patient has an amputation, if the patient places excessive body weight toward the rear of the wheelchair, or if the patient has a history of tipping wheelchairs backward (Figure 6-1D).

Indications

- LE amputations
- Low patient mass in front of wheelchair or high mass in rear
- History of tipping wheelchair backward

Disadvantages

- Larger turning radius because frame base is longer.[3]
- Based on SCI studies, chairs with the rear wheels moved posteriorly can negatively affect propulsion performance.[9]

One-Hand Drive

One-hand-drive wheelchairs or mechanisms permit self-propulsion and steering using only one upper extremity. Two wheel rims attach to only one side of the frame;[10] pushing one rim permits the wheelchair to steer left while pushing the other rim allows the wheelchair to steer right. Pushing both rims simultaneously allows the wheelchair to go straight. The patient therefore needs to have well-coordinated hand function on one side to operate this mechanism. Patients may assume an undesirable asymmetrical trunk posture by leaning toward the handrim when operating the one-hand-drive mechanism. Based on clinical experience, it may also place added stress onto one side of the frame if the patient chronically leans over to the side during propulsion (Figure 6-1E).

Indications

- Stroke patients
- Self-propulsion using an uninvolved UE

Disadvantages

- Difficulty to grasp and operate one-hand drives
- Patients tend to assume an asymmetric posture

Mobility Bases for Orientation in Space

Backward Tilt-in-Space Frames

Backward tilt-in-space frames tilt posteriorly in space like a rocking chair, except the position of the frame can be adjusted and maintained at various angles while the hips are maintained at a fixed angle. As a result, the patient's posture can be varied from upright sitting with the patient facing front to fully tilted backward with the patient facing up toward the ceiling. Manufacturers offer various tilt designs (e.g., fixed pivot point, curved gears) that in turn can have an impact on the chair's length and patient's weight distribution in the chair.

Backward tilt-in-space frames should be considered if patients need pressure relief, have poor head control or poor trunk control, or tend to slide forward in the wheelchair, because gravity can assist sitting. Head support is required for this frame when the patient is in backward tilt (Figures 6-4A and 6-5).

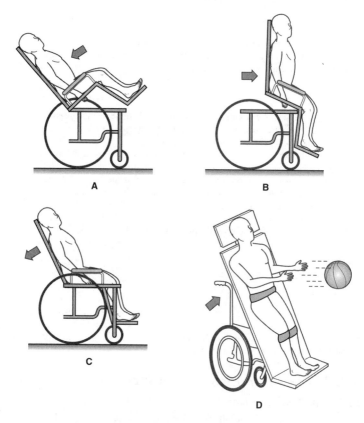

A

B

C

D

FIGURE 6-4 A variety of mobility bases address orientation in space. **(A)** Backward tilt-in-space frames permit gravity-assisted sitting for patients with poor sitting ability or sliding problems while the patient's hip joint angles as well as the angle between the seat and back are kept constant. **(B)** Forward tilt-in-space frames allow the patient to be tipped forward if a more up-right position is needed. **(C)** Reclining frames may be appropriate for patients with poor head control, poor sitting tolerance, or hip extension contractures. **(D)** Standing mobility offers the patient interaction with the environment from a standing rather than sitting posture.

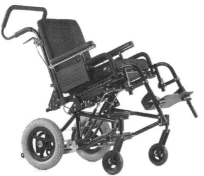

Ischial Pressure Reduction and Backward Tilt

The evidence is compelling that backward tilt offers some pressure relief. In a meta-analysis of five studies involving neurologic populations, Michael et al. reported that interface pressures under the ischia decreased about 24 mm Hg (24.0 [95% CI 4.19–43.8 mm Hg]) using backward tilt angles between 20 and 45 degrees.[11] Henderson et al. found that a 65-degree backward tilt significantly reduced ischial pressure an average of 47% in 10 persons with SCI (7 paraplegia, 3 tetraplegia), although only 1 of the 10 persons achieved a pressure below 32 mm Hg.[12] A 35-degree backward tilt failed to reduce sitting pressures statistically. Finally, Hobson found that in 12 active but complete SCI wheelchair users (5 tetraplegia, 7 paraplegia; age 25–66 years), maximal sitting pressures were reduced 11% when users were placed in a 20-degree backward tilt compared with a neutral upright sitting position (with back slightly opened to a 100-degree recline).[13] He estimated that a 25-degree backward tilt position would result in a 100% reduction in shear force.

Disadvantages for backward tilt include sensory deprivation/isolation due to the patient facing more or less toward the ceiling when the frame is tilted backward. The frame is also heavier, larger, and more costly than a standard frame. Finally, it folds, by collapsing the back posts forward onto the seat, into a less compact size than a standard frame.

Indications (Also See Indications for Power Seating)

- Pressure reduction[11–13]
- Poor head control
- Poor trunk control
- Forward sliding in wheelchair
- Poor tolerance for upright sitting
- Instability of head and trunk during transportation[10]

Disadvantages

- Heavier and larger than standard frame
- Folding is possible but less compact
- Sensory deprivation/isolation
- Cost

Reclining Frame (Semi- and Full Reclining)

Reclining frames permit the back to be reclined like a lawn chair and should be considered if patients have poor head control, cannot tolerate an upright position (need sitting pressure reduction), or have hip extension contractures. Head support is required for this frame when the patient is reclined (Figures 6-4C and Figure 6-6).

Reclining frames can reduce sitting pressures. Hobson found that in 12 active but complete SCI wheelchair users (5 tetraplegia, 7 paraplegia; ages 25–66 years) maximal sitting pressures were reduced up to 12% while in a 120-degree recline position; however, recline also led to a 25% rise in shear forces.[13]

The reclining frame has some disadvantages. First, contact points between the patient's back and the back support of the wheelchair do not remain consistent when the back angle is changed using a traditional recliner mechanism. Instead, contact points move up cephalically as the frame reclines. As a result, patients may tend to slide forward with shear forces created between the patient's backside and the reclining back of the wheelchair.[14] Also, if lateral trunk supports are attached, they will tend to ride up into the patient's axilla with increased recline angles. Second, sensory deprivation/isolation may occur when the patient faces up toward the ceiling once the back is reclined. Third, the reclined position may facilitate undesirable extensor tone in neurological patients caused by tonic labyrinthine reflex (TLR) activation.[15] Finally, reclining frames are heavier and larger than standard wheelchair frames.

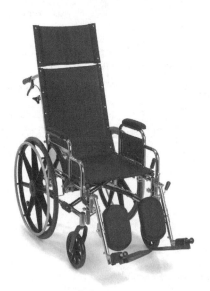

FIGURE 6-6 Reclining frame. (Courtesy of Sunrise Medical)

Indications (Also See Indications for Power Seating)

- If lacking 90 degrees of hip flexion
- Poor head control
- Poor trunk control
- Moderate trunk involvement—semi-reclining[16]
- Severe trunk involvement—full reclining[16]
- Comfort/unable to tolerate upright sitting

Disadvantages

- Shear is present (nonshear recline systems are available but are more expensive)[14]
- Sensory deprivation/isolation (i.e., the patient faces the ceiling)
- Heavier and larger than standard frame
- TLR may increase extensor tone

Forward Tilt-in-Space Frame

Forward tilt-in-space frames actually tilt or pitch the patient forward as if someone lifted the back legs of the chair you were sitting on. This frame should be considered if it is important for the patient to be upright but lacks the hip range to do so. For example, an individual may choke if fed in a reclined position but lacks adequate hip flexion to sit upright in a standard wheelchair. The forward tilt therefore enables the patient's body to be pitched forward as one unit. The disadvantage of this frame is that the patient will tend to slide forward in the wheelchair. These frames are also costlier, heavier, and larger than a standard frame (Figure 6-4B).

Indications

- Unable to tolerate a reclined position
- LE extension contractures

Disadvantages

- Forward sliding/shear associated with sliding
- Heavier and larger than standard frame
- Cost

Elevating and Standing Mobility

Elevating chairs are powered and enable seat height to be raised and lowered[14] to facilitate functional reach and enhance social interaction (see Figure 6-13). Standing mobility enables patients to interact from a supported standing position if sufficient LE range of motion is available (Figure 6-4D, 6-14).

Advantages

- Improve reach from different heights[14]
- Social interaction at eye level
- Weight-bearing (standing mobility)
- Alternative positioning (standing mobility)

Disadvantages

- Any contraindications for standing (standing mobility)
- Requires sufficient hip extension, knee extension, and ankle dorsiflexion (standing mobility)
- Cost
- Storage/portability
- Maintenance, if powered
- Safety concerns related to falls from standing or elevated seated positions

Dependent Push Systems (Attendant-Operated Mobility Bases)

Strollers

Strollers are a lightweight means of transportation for infants and small children who do not self-propel. The advantage of a stroller is less weight and greater portability. As a result, parents can get around town, into stores, and up stairs with less difficulty using a stroller than using a wheelchair (Figure 6-7B).

Strollers, however, don't provide as much postural support as would a wheelchair unless you build support into the stroller (which would then increase the weight). The big drawback of strollers is that the patient can't push a stroller because the wheels are small. Growth adjustability in the stroller may also be limited. (Typically, strollers are outgrown by the time the child reaches 4 years old or weighs 40 lbs.)[17] Parents may prefer a stroller to a wheelchair because they feel their child looks less disabled in the stroller. These parents should be aware that the child's independence will be restricted if self-propulsion ability is possible.

Advantages

- Infants
- Lightweight transportation
- Accessibility in the community
- Portability
- Cosmetics—less stigma than wheelchair

Disadvantages

- Can't self-propel
- Less sturdy than a wheelchair

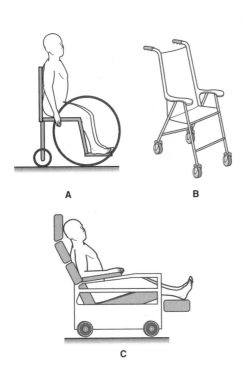

Figure 6-7 Dependent push systems (attendant-operated mobility bases). **(A)** Indoor chairs can be spotted by their larger front wheels and their ability to be maneuvered in tight indoor spaces. **(B)** A stroller offers a lightweight, portable means of transporting a child who does not self-propel; growth capability, postural support, and durability, however, may be less in a stroller than in a wheelchair. **(C)** Geriatric chairs offer the nonambulatory patient a padded, reclined positioning with elevating leg support for indoor use.

- Less postural support options
- Less growth capability

Transport Chairs and Transport Systems

Transport chairs (a wheelchair frame with four small wheels) for adults (Figure 6-8) and transport systems for children who weigh more than 40 lbs may be useful for those who need a portable chair for short trips.[17] Transport systems are generally lighter than standard wheelchairs, cosmetically more acceptable, and easier to manage in narrow hallways and for car storage. These chairs, however, are typically not used for long bouts of sitting during the day. Features to look for in a transport system include foldability, height adjustability, flip-away footrests, postural support, acceptable push handle height, lightness in weight, and growth and tilt capabilities (if needed).[17] For public transportation, make sure the chair/ system is WC-19 compliant and crash tested.[18,19]

FIGURE 6-8 Transport chair. (Courtesy of Sunrise Medical)

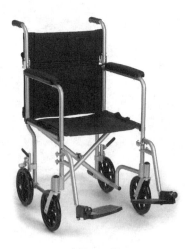

Indoor Chairs

Indoor chairs have large wheels in front and casters in the rear, enabling the wheelchair to be maneuvered in tight areas[3] (Figure 6-7A). Outdoor use is not recommended because curbs and stair negotiation will be difficult due to the wheel configuration. Self-propulsion is possible, but may be more challenging in an indoor chair than in a standard chair.[3]

Indications

- Indoor use
- Small spaces

Disadvantages

- May be difficult to self-propel[3]
- Not for outdoor use
- Difficulty using on curbs and stairs[3]

Geriatric Chairs

Geriatric chairs are mostly seen in facilities for older adults and allow the individual to recline with feet elevated. Disadvantages include limited outdoor use, no ability to self-propel, difficulty for caregiver to steer and push, difficulty to position patients, and difficulty performing two-person transfers. Use may also result in less social interaction (Figure 6-7C).[20]

Indications
- Back recline and foot elevation needed
- Indoor use

Disadvantages
- Patient can't self-propel
- Difficulty transferring
- Difficult for caregiver to push
- Insufficient postural support
- Not for outdoor use
- Sensory deprivation when patient is reclined

Alternative Manual Wheelchairs: Crank and Lever

Although handrim manual wheelchairs are popular (90% use) in Western countries and have an indoor advantage for maneuverability, steering, and storage,[21] their efficiency as a machine is quite low (i.e., 10%).[22] Alternative mobility devices using hand cranks or levers are more popular in other regions of the world and have a number of outdoor advantages including greater efficiency (higher maximal mechanical efficiency, higher top speeds), and less strain (lower cardiovascular strain, lower musculoskeletal strain) as compared to handrim devices (Figure 6-9). Hand crank wheelchairs, however, are too large for indoor use.[21]

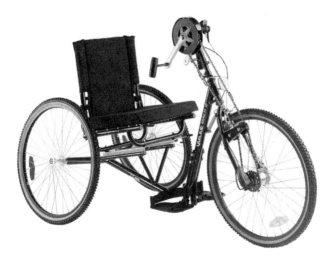

THE MOBILITY BASE

FIGURE 6-9 A hand crank mobility device. (Courtesy of Sunrise Medical)

Power Mobility Device (PMD) Bases

Power mobility devices use a battery to power and operate a mobility base. There are numerous ways to classify power mobility, such as by mobility base (traditional vs. platform); use (indoor vs. outdoor); drive system (rear vs. mid vs. front wheel; direct vs. belt), and portability (rigid vs. folding). The Centers for Medicare and Medicaid Services (CMS) recently developed 64 codes for power mobility devices, contained within categories that span from devices for light duty/part-day use to devices for full-time/active use. The categories are: light use, consumer rehab, complex rehab, high-activity use, pediatric, and miscellaneous (such as pushrim-activated, power-assisted wheelchair [PAPAW] and add-on conversion kits). Within each category, products are further differentiated by seat type (sling, caption, solid), weight capacity (standard, up to 300 lb; heavy duty, up to 450 lb; very heavy duty, to 600 lb; extra heavy duty, >600 lb) and power feature options (single power [e.g., tilt functions] or multiple power [e.g., tilt and recliner or ventilator functions]).[22]

In this section, various power mobility devices will be reviewed (Figure 6-10).

Add-on Power System

Add-on power systems convert an existing manual wheelchair into a power chair.[13] They may be indicated for manual wheelchair owners with a need for power mobility but limited funding. The disadvantage is less durable power mobility.

Pushrim-Activated Power-Assisted Wheelchairs (PAPAW)

Pushrim-activated power-assisted wheelchairs (PAPAW) are relatively new in the market and may serve as a compromise between manual and power mobility (Figure 6-11). By activating small motors via the handrims of the wheelchair, the user experiences a small burst of propulsion power that can aid in negotiations of ramps, uneven terrain (carpet), and distant outdoor destinations. It may also help reduce the UE biomechanical stresses in users with UE pathology associated with manual wheelchair use (i.e., in persons with spinal cord injuries).[23,24]

Cooper et al. reported less energy demand (O_2 consumption and heart rate) in 10 wheelchair users (9 paraplegia, 1 multiple sclerosis [MS]) propelling a PAPAW at two speeds (1.8 and 0.9 m/s) on a treadmill when compared with their own chairs.[25] Best et al. studied young adult nonwheelchair users' preference for PAPAW versus lightweight manual chairs during various wheelchair tasks.[26] Interestingly, volunteers indicated a preference for PAPAW when performing torque-required skills (curbs, inclines, and irregular [gravel] surfaces), but a preference for the manual wheelchair when more control was required (e.g., wheelies, turns, door opening, and parallel parking). Generalizability of the findings is limited because volunteers were able-bodied.

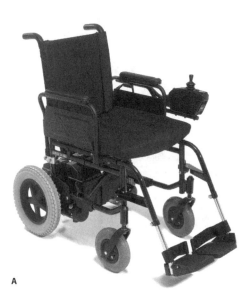

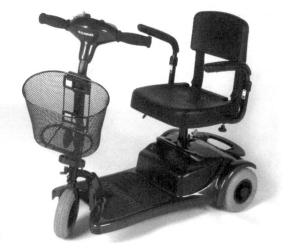

FIGURE 6-10 Power mobility bases. **(A)** A folding, lightweight power wheelchair is the traditional model of power mobility that offers postural support for patients who cannot self-propel a manual wheelchair. **(B)** Scooters look like golf carts and offer power mobility for the patient with limited endurance but sufficient sitting, transfer, and UE (steering) ability. (Courtesy of Sunrise Medical)

A

B

THE MOBILITY BASE

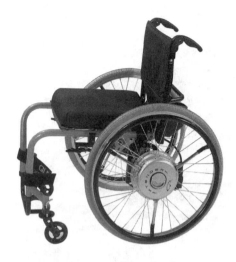

FIGURE 6-11 Pushrim-activated power-assisted wheelchair. (Courtesy of Sunrise Medical)

Disadvantages

- Added weight (additional 50+ lbs) due primarily to the batteries
- Difficulty pushing in an inactivated mode (i.e., when battery dies)
- Cost and funding issues
- May be more difficult to remove and reinsert wheels[26]
- Some wheelchair activities like wheelies and ascending curbs may be more difficult to execute.[26]

Power-Operated Vehicles (POVs) (Scooters)

Power-operated vehicles are motorized carts that use a tiller (bar; lever) to steer. POVs generally require better sitting ability, transfer ability, and manual upper limb (steering wheel) ability than do patients using a power wheelchair (Figure 6-10B). Patients may be marginal ambulators.[3,14] Scooters can have three or four wheels and are lighter and narrower than power wheelchairs. In addition, less of a stigma may be attached to a cart than a power wheelchair.[3] Be cautious about recommending a scooter to a patient who has a progressive disability and may soon lack the transfer, upper extremity function, or postural control needed to use one. In this case, a power wheelchair may be more appropriate.[27] Scooter selection is based in part on whether it will be used indoors, outdoors, or both indoors and outdoors.[28]

Indications

- Ambulation and manual wheelchair propulsion difficulties
- Limited stamina[27] (e.g., post polio, cardiac patient)
- Good transfer skills, sitting balance, and UE function

Advantages[10]

- Lighter in weight than a power wheelchair
- Narrower than a power wheelchair
- Looks less handicapping than a power wheelchair

Disadvantages

- Maintenance
- Cost
- Inaccessibility
- Requires adequate UE, sitting, and transfer abilities
- Lacks portability/folding/storage (some can be disassembled)
- Lacks postural support
- Stability problems—incidence of tipping over

Power Wheelchairs (Electric Wheelchairs)

Power wheelchair mobility can offer independence for patients who can safely operate the controls, cannot manually self-propel a wheelchair, and require postural support (Figure 6-10A).[29] Patients may be marginal manual wheelchair users.[3,14] Social, cognitive, perceptual, and functional developmental benefits of using power mobility have been reported in physically disabled children as young as 24 months.[14] Control type (i.e., operating switches) and placement will be critical to evaluate for patient independence. (Also see Chapter 4, Power Mobility Evaluations.)

Indications

- Independent mobility possible using power but not manual wheelchair or POV (scooter)
- High tetraplegia/permanent disability
- Physical exertion is contraindicated
- Marginal manual wheelchair user—unable to maintain appropriate rate of locomotion in manual wheelchair[14]
- For energy conservation[14]

Disadvantages

- Accessibility problems
- Cost (three times more costly than manual wheelchair)
- Back-up manual wheelchair needed[28] (some funding sources may not pay for two wheelchairs)[30]
- Portability/folding/storage is difficult or lacking
- Heavy (battery adds weight)
- Maintenance

Both power wheelchairs and scooters require routine battery charging. Neither fair well in inaccessible neighborhoods where curb cuts, ramps, and beveled sidewalks are absent. Both are heavier than manual wheelchairs, which makes getting up one step with assistance difficult and getting up more than one step nearly impossible. In addition, if a power wheelchair or scooter breaks down, it's much heavier to push home than a manual wheelchair. (It's a little like pushing a car in neutral as compared with a bicycle.) Consider a manual wheelchair (or transport chair) as a backup in case the power wheelchair needs to go to the shop for repairs. (However, keep in mind that not all funding sources will pay for two chairs).[30]

Control Interface

Switches, which control the chair's locomotion, as well as other features, can provide either on/off or graded operations.[10] The control parameters may be either fixed (nonprogrammable, factory settings) or have varying levels of programmability (tailoring to the balance and reflex needs of the user).[31] These features can regulate speed, acceleration, direction, and sensitivity (e.g., damping for tremors). Electronic controls also can be used to operate power tilt and/or recline features. Attendant drive controls also are available and may be useful for attendant-assisted operation.[32] Be aware that too many control features may place excessive perceptual motor demands on some patients.[33]

- *Proportional controls*—Offer gradation in speed and change in direction as the control switch moves away from its center (see Figure 6-10A). An analogous device would be the accelerator in a car, where the greater the physical displacement of the pedal, the greater the acceleration.[34] Another example is the dimmer light switch in a room. Graded (proportional) switches therefore offer patients more control over wheelchair operations. Examples of proportional control interfaces include *conventional joysticks*, finger and mini joysticks, and pads. Because proportional joysticks require patient movement, some joint proprioception and joint mobility is required.

   Conventional joysticks may require greater force to activate as compared with other controls. In an observational study, Pellegrini et al. found 18 adults with advanced Duchenne Muscular Dystrophy (DMD) who were evaluated for new switches on their power chairs were able to progress from restricted to unrestricted power wheelchair use after being provided alternative joystick switches, which required less activating forces.[35]

- *Isometric controls*—Can offer gradation of wheelchair response using graded muscle force rather than displacement. An analogous device would be the "eraser head mouse" used on some laptop computers.[34] Isometric joysticks may require less strength (and joint movement) from the user, but because they require the use of graded force, the control interface may be too sensitive for persons with tremor or spasticity.

- *Microswitch controls*—Provide on/off operation for patients with limited motor ability. Microswitch controls require no gradation from the user. An analogous device would be the light switch in a room—it's either on or off, no in-between. A microswitch example is a sip and puff control used to activate a power wheelchair by a person with high-level tetraplegia.[34]

Drive Wheel Configurations

The drive wheel for power chairs can be located in the rear, middle, or front of the frame (i.e., the wheel that drives the chair).

The location of the drive wheel can affect wheelchair performance.[31,36]

Rear Wheel Drive (RWD)
Drive wheel is located behind the user/the chair pushes (Figure 6-10A). [31,36]

- Traditional/original design good for rural settings
- No fishtailing (rear swerving) at high speeds
- Large turning radius leads to difficulty maneuvering in small spaces
- Better traction uphill compared to downhill

Front Wheel Drive (FWD)
Drive wheel is in front of user/the chair pulls.[31,36]

- Small turning radius for maneuvering in small spaces
- Better traction downhill compared to uphill
- Top speeds are limited—rear of chair swerves (fishtails) at high speeds

Mid-Wheel Drive (MWD)
Drive wheel is under patient—most recent design (Figure 6-12).[31,36]

- Best for indoor use—smallest turning radius for maneuvering in small spaces. Turning may be more intuitive using a mid-drive configuration (i.e., drive wheels beneath the user). In a case report of a power chair evaluation for a

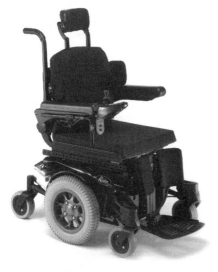

FIGURE 6-12 Mid-wheel drive power chair. (Courtesy of Sunrise Medical)

12-year-old child with cerebral palsy, Huhn et al.[36] described the success the child experienced in negotiating turns in the home (better furniture clearance) once she switched from a rear- to a mid-drive chair.[36]

- Provides traction uphill and downhill
- Difficulties ascending curbs or turning on uneven ground (e.g., grass)

Four Wheel Drive
Good for outdoor use and extreme conditions/traction needs.

- Is expensive, heavier, and has a larger turning radius

Power Features: Tilt/Recline/Passive Standing/Elevation/ Stair Climbing Systems

Power chairs can also be equipped with features to change body orientation, or height, or even to climb stairs. Power tilt and/or recline can be used to alter sitting pressure distribution by changing chair orientation. Power elevation can facilitate reaching for high shelves (e.g., at the grocery store), adjusting seat height to optimize transfer position (i.e., sliding type), and socializing (talking face to face) (Figure 6-13). Power standing features offer passive weight-bearing experiences through the lower extremities, bladder emptying, and pressure relief from sitting (Figure 6-14).[37] The advantages of power stair-climbing systems are obvious, although use of a stair rail or the presence of a caregiver may be required based on company protocol and driving tests (Figure 6-15).[38] Other power options abound, including power flip-back armrests and power flip-foot platforms to facilitate transfers.[39]

Patient Preferences for Power Tilt/Recline

Popular patient preferences and uses for power tilt/recline do not necessarily match well-known medical indications. In a random Canadian sample of interviewed adult power tilt/recline users with varying diagnoses (e.g., MS, neuromuscular disease, SCI), Lacoste et al. found the top reasons for using tilt/recline were *comfort, rest,* and *bladder management.*[40] More users used a tilt instead of a recliner for sliding problems whereas the opposite was true for bladder and respiration management. Curiously, pressure relief was low on users' lists.

Indications for Power Seating: Tilt and/or Recline[22,41]

- High risk for pressure ulcers and not able to weight shift
- To manage spasticity/tone
- Intermittent catheterization required and not able to transfer independently from power chair to bed

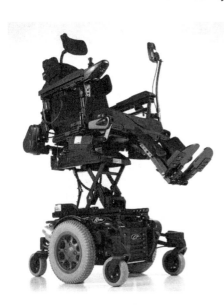

FIGURE 6-13 (left) Power chair with elevation feature. (Courtesy of Sunrise Medical)

FIGURE 6-14 (bottom left) Power chair with standing feature. (Courtesy of Permobil, Inc.)

FIGURE 6-15 (bottom right) Power chair with stair climbing feature. (Courtesy of Independence Technology)

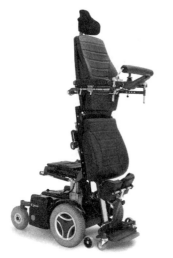

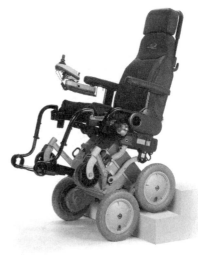

THE MOBILITY BASE

Power Frame Types[31]

- *Folding*—Portable for car transportation, but chair must be disassembled and battery removed (Figure 6-10A).
- *Rigid*—Durable, but generally requires van or truck transportation due to storage problem (Figure 6-12).

Power Wheelchairs and ANSI/RESNA Wheelchair Standards

Power chair safety and performance testing outcomes appear to vary for both low-cost and higher grade models. Pearlman et al. compared a few low-cost, nonprogrammable power chairs ($n = 3$; each with a captain's chair) from different manufacturers using the ANSI/RESNA wheelchair standards and found variation in both safety (static tipping) and reliability results (system failures, fatigue tests).[42] Rentschler et al. compared a few higher grade (more expensive) power wheelchairs ($n = 5$) from different manufacturers using the ANSI/RESNA wheelchair standards and found that performance varied with regard to stability, strength, climatic conditioning, energy consumption, and braking distance.[43] In both studies, the number of models tested was limited.

The Future: Smart Wheelchairs

Smart wheelchairs, a term to describe either robotics with an added seat or alternatively a power wheelchair with computer sensors, have been under development to address a segment of the disabled community for whom conventional power mobility is not an option due to visual, cognitive, or motor (spasticity/tremor) deficits. These devices can operate under a number of modes including autonomous navigation, collision avoidance, wall following, passage through doors, and traveling to targets. Although they can operate indoors, outdoor challenges (e.g., drop offs), costs/insurance coverage, and liability have limited their commercial use.[44]

The future challenge will be to interface advancements in robotics, artificial intelligence, and other technologies with the human factor so people with significant disabilities can negotiate outdoor (stairs, weather) and indoor (tight space) environments.[45]

EXERCISE

Go to the Internet and get a ballpark price range for the following mobility bases: strollers, manual wheelchairs (standard, lightweight, ultralight, recliner, tilt-in-space) and power mobility (scooter, power wheelchair).

References

1. Cooper RA, Gonzalez J, Lawrence B, Renschler A, Boninger ML, VanSickle DP. Performance of selected lightweight wheelchairs on ANSI/RESNA tests. American National Standards Institute, Rehabilitation Engineering and Assistive Technology Society of North America. *Arch Phys Med Rehabil.* 1997;78(10):1138–1144.
2. Cooper RA, Robertson RN, Lawrence B, et al. Life-cycle analysis of depot versus rehabilitation manual wheelchairs. *J Rehabil Res Dev.* 1996;33(1):45–55.
3. Wilson AB, Mcfarland SR. Types of wheelchairs. *J Rehabil Res Dev.* 1990;2(Supp):104–116.
4. Ragnarsson KT. Clinical perspectives on wheelchair selection: prescription considerations and a comparison of conventional and light weight wheelchairs. *J Rehabil Res Dev.* 1990;2(Supp):8–16.
5. Parziale JR. Standard v lightweight wheelchair propulsion in spinal cord injured patients. *Am J Phys Med Rehabil.* 1991;70(2):76–80.
6. Paleg G. Not a lightweight decision. *Rehab Manag.* 2007;(3):26–29.
7. Beekman CE, Miller-Porter L, Schoneberger M. Energy cost of propulsion in standard and ultralight wheelchairs in people with spinal cord injuries. *Phys Ther.* 1999;79(2):146–158.
8. Cooper RA, Boninger ML, Rentschler A. Evaluation of selected ultralight manual wheelchairs using ANSI/RESNA standards. *Arch Phys Med Rehabil.* 1999;80(4):462–467.
9. Boninger ML, Baldwin M, Cooper RA, Koontz A, Chan L. Manual wheelchair pushrim biomechanics and axle position. *Arch Phys Med Rehabil.* 2000;81(5):608–613.
10. Harrymann SE, Warren LR. Positioning and power mobility. In: Church G, Glennen S, eds. *The Handbook of Assistive Technologies.* San Diego: Singular; 1992:55–92.
11. Michael SM, Porter D, Pountney TE. Tilted seat position for non-ambulant individuals with neurological and neuromuscular impairment: a systematic review. *Clini Rehabil.* 2007;21:1063–1074.
12. Henderson JL, Price SH, Brandstater ME, Mandac BR. Efficacy of three measures to relieve pressure in seated persons with spinal cord injury. *Arch Phys Med Rehabil.* 1994;75:535–539.
13. Hobson DA. Comparative effects of posture on pressure and shear at the body-seat interface. *J Rehabil Res & Dev.* 1992;29(4):21–31.
14. Warren CG. Technical considerations: power mobility and its implications. *J Rehabil Res Dev* 1990;2(Supp):44–85.
15. Fiorentino MR. *Reflex Testing Methods for Evaluating CNS Development*, 2nd ed. Springfield IL: Charles C Thomas; 1981:17.
16. Delisa JA, Greenberg S. Wheelchair prescription guidelines. *Am Fam Physician* 1982;24:145–150.
17. Paleg G. The right fit. *Rehab Manag.* 2003;16(2):26–28, 31.
18. Paleg G. A proper position. Determining the appropriate seating and positioning for transporting the pediatric client. *Rehab Manag.* 2007;20(7):16, 18, 20.

THE MOBILITY BASE

19. Paleg G. Push, propel, or stroll? Advice on choosing the perfect system for very young children. *Rehab Manage.* 2006;19(5):40, 42, 44–45.

20. Sabol TP, Haley ES. Wheelchair evaluation for the older adult *Clin Geriatr Med.* 2006;22:355–375.

21. Van der Woude LHV, Dallmeijer AJ, Janssen TWJ, et al. Alternative modes of manual wheelchair ambulation: an overview. *Am J Phys Med Rehabil.* 2001;80:765–777.

22. Paleg G. Subject to approval. Available at: http://www.rehabpub.com/issues/articles/2007-01_04.asp. Accessed October 29, 2008.

23. Karmarkar A, Cooper RA, Liu H, Connor S, Puhlman J. Evaluation of pushrim-activated power-assisted wheelchairs using ANSI/RESNA standards. *Arch Phys Med Rehabil.* 2008;89:1191–1198.

24. Levy CE, Chow JW. Pushrim-activated power-assist wheelchairs: elegance in motion. *Am J Phys Med Rehabil.* 2004;83(2):166–167.

25. Cooper RA, Fitzgerald SG, Boninger ML, et al. Evaluation of a pushrim-activated, power-assisted wheelchair. *Arch Phys Med Rehabil.* 2001;82:702–708.

26. Best KL, Kirby RL, Smith C, Macleod DA. Comparison between performance with a pushrim-activated power-assisted wheelchair and a manual wheelchair on the wheelchair skills test. *Disability Rehabil.* 2006;28(4):213–220.

27. Currie DM, Hardwick K, Marburger RA, Britell CW. Wheelchair prescription and adaptive seating. In Delisa JL, Gans BM, eds. *Rehabilitation Medicine: Principles and Practice.* 2nd ed. Philadelphia: J B Lippincott; 1993:563–585.

28. Rivette CM, personal communication, October 3, 1997.

29. Miles-Tapping C, MacDonald LJ. Lifestyle implications of power mobility. *Phys Occup Ther Geriatr.* 1994;12:31–49.

30. Canning B. Funding ethics, and assistive technology: should medical necessity be the criterion by which wheeled mobility equipment is justified? *Top Stroke Rehabil.* 2005;12(3):77.

31. Tieszen LM, Johnston TG. The power of selection. Available at: http://www.rehabpub.com/ltrehab/42001/4.asp. Accessed October 29, 2008.

32. Cohen D. Optional but necessary. *Rehab Manag.* 2005;18(10):26, 28–29.

33. Batavia M, Batavia AI, Friedman R. Changing chairs: anticipating problems in prescribing wheelchairs. *Disability Rehabil.* 2001;23(12):539–548.

34. Dicianno BE, Spaeth DM, Cooper RA, Fitzgerald SG, Boninger ML. Advancements in power wheelchair joystick technology: effects of isometric joysticks and signal conditioning on driving performance. *Am J Phys Med Rehabil.* 2006;85(8):631–639.

35. Pellegrini N, Guillon B, Prigent H, et al. Optimization of power wheelchair control for patients with severe Duchenne muscular dystrophy. *Neuromuscular Disord.* 2004;14:297–300.

36. Huhn K, Guarrera-Bowlby P, Deutsch JE. The clinical decision-making process of prescribing power mobility for a child with cerebral palsy. *Pediatr Phys Ther.* 2007;19(3):254–260.

37. Edlich RF, Winters KL, Nelson KP, et al. Technological advances in power wheelchairs. *J Long Term Eff Med Implants.* 2004;14(2):107–129.

38. Independence Technology. *iBOT Your Life: Independence iBot Mobility System.* [Brochure]. Binghamton, NY: Johnson & Johnson; 2008.

39. Paleg G. What's new in mobility accessories. *Rehab Manage.* 2007;20(2):24, 26–27.

40. Lacoste M, Weiss-Lambrou RW, Allard M, Dansereau J. Powered tilt/recline systems: why and how are they used? *Asst Technol.* 2003;15:58–68.

41. Dicianno BE, Tovey E. Power mobility device provision: understanding Medicare guidelines and advocating for clients. *Arch Phys Med Rehabil.* 2007;88:807–816.

42. Pearlman JL, Cooper RA, Karnawat J, Cooper R, Boninger ML. Evaluation of the safety and durability of low-cost nonprogrammable electric powered wheelchairs. *Arch Phys Med Rehabil.* 2005;86(12):2361–2370.

43. Rentschler AJ, Cooper RA, Fitzgerald SG, et al. Evaluation of selected electric-powered wheelchairs using the ANSI/RESNA standards. *Arch Phys Med Rehabil.* 2004;85(4):611–619.

44. Simpson RC. Smart wheelchairs: a literature review. *J Rehabil Res Devel.* 2005;42(4):423–436.

45. Cooper RA, Ding D, Grindle GG, Wang H. Personal mobility and manipulation using robotics, artificial intelligence, and advanced control. Proceedings of the 29th Annual International Conference of the IEEE EMBS in Lyon, France; August 23–26, 2007.

THE MOBILITY BASE

CHAPTER 7

Seating System and Wheelchair Components

Shopping for wheelchair parts is a little like buying a computer. All options (speed, size, memory, cost, appearance) for each component (hard drive, printer, monitor, CPU, modem) need to be carefully considered so your personal needs are met. For wheelchair components, many options also exist. The supplier will help you configure "your system" once you know what you want. When possible, consider less costly commercially available parts that will sufficiently address the patient's needs. The most common wheelchair components, including seating system components, will be reviewed in this chapter. (Note: Throughout this chapter alternative terminology will be provided in parentheses.)

Commercial Versus Custom-Made Components

Commercially Available

- Available
- Less costly
- Less tailored to specific needs
- Returnable

Custom-Made

- More costly
- Not returnable
- More time to fabricate
- Specific to patient's special needs

Headrest

The headrest (head support[1]) is a support structure on the wheelchair located behind the patient's head (Figure 7-1).

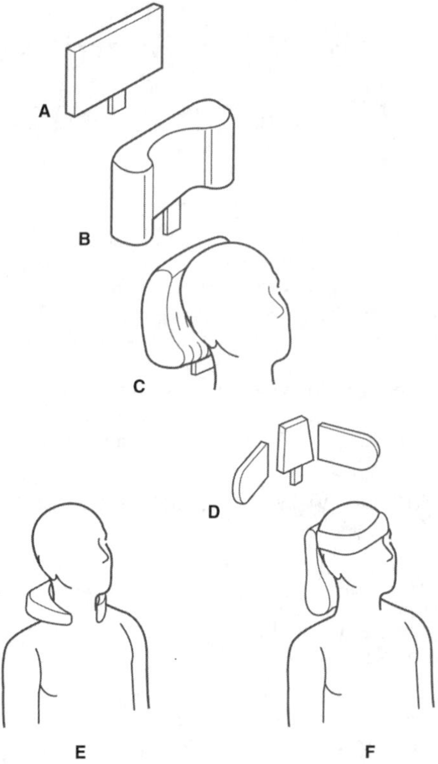

FIGURE 7-1 Types of head supports: **(A)** planar, **(B)** curve, **(C)** curved headrest with occipital support, **(D)** central and side panels, **(E)** neck ring, **(F)** head band.

Indications

- Difficulty maintaining head upright
- Support for the head while in a reclined or backward tilt position[2]
- Protect against whiplash injury during bus or van transportation

Disadvantages

- May interfere with two-person transfers; consider removable headrests
- Adds weight to the wheelchair

Types

Head support shapes are *planar (flat)* or *curved* depending on how much contact is needed between the patient's head and the headrest.

Comments

- Consider a *planar headrest* if the patient needs support primarily behind the head.

- Consider a *curved headrest* if the patient needs lateral support for the head (i.e., head falls to the side; see Figure 6-13). Side panels can provide additional lateral support.

- Consider an *occipital support/ledge* to cradle the head (where the neck and back of the head meet) if the patient has sufficient occipital contact points (Figures E-3B2 and E-3B3). The support can be built into the shape of the headrest. Although an occipital ledge can provide cervical support in flexion, some patients may respond by pushing back against the headrest with undesirable scapula elevation.[3]

- Headrests can affect head position, muscle tone, neck position, and swallowing ability.[4]

- If the patient presents with strong extensor tone or activity, consider a reinforced, stronger headrest system.

- If the patient tends to hook the head around the side of the headrest, consider a wider headrest or deep headrest with lateral walls (side panels) to block the hooking behavior.

- If the headrest is too high (i.e., above the crown of the head) it may block the vision of the attendant helping with propulsion and may interfere with clearance in low-roof vans.

- If the headrest is too wide (i.e., extends beyond the ears), it may block the patient's view behind the wheelchair.

- If the side panels of a headrest are too narrow (i.e., less than ear-to-ear width), irritation of the ears, temporal mandibular joint (TMJ), or lateral corner of the eye may result from friction and rubbing.

- *Neck collars/rings* (i.e., cervical supports attached to the wheelchair) may help maintain the patient's head in an erect position[5] and keep the neck centered.[3]

- *Head bands* (i.e., bands attached to the headrest that provide anterior support around the patient's forehead) have been used to position the patient's head back into the postural support structure.[3] These head support structures have been used by some patients who lack head control but need to function from an upright position.

- *Caution is required for any devices used around the head and neck.* Items used around the patient's head and neck should be evaluated carefully and supervised adequately due to risk of injury. Patients who slide forward in their wheelchair or are poorly positioned can get hung up on these devices. Devices around the head can affect tone, swallowing, and posture.[4]

- Try to provide the least restrictive environment with the minimal amount of restraints to achieve the goals of sitting. One strategy is to provide gravity-assisted support (tilt-in-space or reclining wheelchair) to minimize the patient's reliance on anterior head and trunk supports.

Back Support/Insert

The back support structures on the wheelchair can range from simple fabric/ upholstery support to inserts with a firm base and a padded contact surface.

Back insert shapes are *planar* or *curved (contoured)* depending on how much material is needed to maximize contact with the patient's back. The more severe a fixed deformity or asymmetry, the greater the need for contoured support (Figure 7-2).

Advantage

• Provides postural support for the patient's back.

Types of Back Supports

Back support types include sling back, planar, contoured, and custom molded (Figure 7-3).

Sling Back Upholstery

A sling back provides a backrest that is attached to the back posts of the frame and is usually made of vinyl material. It is often the default back support provided by the manufacturer (see Figure 6-8).[3] This type of backrest offers minimal postural support and may cause a hammocking or rounding effect on the patient's back, giving the patient a fetal-like appearance.

Adjustable Tension Back Upholstery

Adjustable tension back upholstery is an alternative fabric back whose straps can be adjusted in tension to provide additional back support and minimize hammocking. However, persons with marked positioning issues will need more equipment.[6]

Linear/Commercial Planar Inserts

These planar (i.e., flat) support structures provide midline stability in mildly involved patients.[4] (See Figure 6-5.)

Indications

• Minimal orthopedic problems
• Sitting ROM is within normal limits (WNL)
• Able to assume upright sitting

Contoured Combined with Linear Insert

These are curved and planar support structures used to both correct and accommodate patient deformities in moderately involved patients.[4] (See Figure 6-15.)

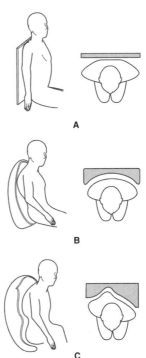

FIGURE 7-2 (right) **(A)** Planar back inserts provide support for mildly involved patients with minimal orthopedic problems. **(B)** Contoured inserts provide support and accommodate deformity in moderately involved patients. **(C)** Custom contoured backs (molded) provides accommodating support for severely involved patients with fixed, asymmetrical deformity.

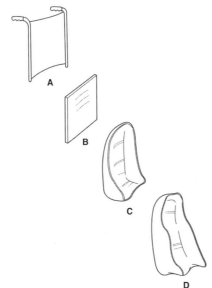

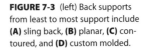

FIGURE 7-3 (left) Back supports from least to most support include **(A)** sling back, **(B)** planar, **(C)** contoured, and **(D)** custom molded.

Indications

- Moderate tone and strength problems
- Moderate orthopedic problems
- Less than 30-degree scoliosis
- Unable to assume symmetrical sitting

Custom Contoured (Molded) Back Inserts

These are curved molded support structures to accommodate deformity in severely involved patients.[4] Clinicians and suppliers need to have experience to produce a good mold.[7] The insert becomes a mirror copy of the back and should fit the patient like a glove, accommodating the hollow and hump-like shape of the patient's spine and rib cage. Custom contoured backs generally provide a tight fit and may interfere with weight-shifting/postural adjustments as well as UE movements in patients who have those abilities. Because a molded insert is cast like a crown for a tooth, it cannot be modified later. Therefore, a molded insert is not recommended if the patient's weight or body shape is likely to change. Although children are candidates for molding, they will require costly periodic replacements due to growth.

Indications

- Severe bony deformity
- Severe tone
- Altered sensation

Disadvantages

- Costly
- Limited growth capability—a distinct disadvantage for children (periodic replacement will be needed)
- Experience needed for successful molding

Comments

- Back inserts add weight to the wheelchair.
- Folding the wheelchair is more difficult. You must remove the back insert prior to folding. Sling-type supports do not encounter this problem.
- The back insert may push the patient too far forward in the wheelchair, making it difficult to reach the wheels during propulsion.[2] Consider an adjustable rear wheel axle to move wheels forward and closer to the upper limbs, or consider hardware to move the back insert further to the rear of the frame if the individual propels the wheelchair.
- Patients who sit well using only the sling back upholstery, or preferably fabric with adjustable tension on the wheelchair, may not require an insert.

- Patients with "relatively" flat backs may benefit from a flat (planar) insert. Some children may fit into this category. Clinicians, however, may argue that because the healthy back exhibits a mild lumbar arch, the back insert should follow the contour of the back rather than offer only planar support.
- Patients with fixed rounded backs, such as geriatric patients with kyphosis, may tolerate or benefit more from accommodating curved (spoon-shaped), commercially available back inserts.
- Patients with severely fixed curvature of the back (scoliosis) may benefit from a custom molded insert.[4]
- The back angle may be reclined 2 to 5 degrees from the vertical[8] because the patient may feel as if they are falling forward if they sit with the back insert installed absolutely vertical.
- Back height is based on the sitting balance requirements and activity level of the patient.[9] A higher back will provide more spinal support but may also limit trunk mobility. A lower back provides less spinal support and may increase risk of spinal deformity and pain, but facilitates the ability to "pop a wheelie."[8] The lumbar spine needs to be supported regardless of back height.[10]
- If a high back height (above the inferior angle of the scapula) is required, consider rounding the top edges of the back insert to free up scapula mobility for less-restricted manual self-propulsion.[8]

Seat Inserts

A seat insert is a support structure usually consisting of a base (i.e., wood, metal, plastic) and cushion.

Types of Seat Inserts

Seat inserts can be *planar (flat), curved, or custom molded* depending on how much contact, support, and pressure distribution is needed between the patient and the seat (Figure 7-4). Sling seat upholstery is not desirable because it provides poor postural support and promotes a hammocking effect resulting in hip adduction, internal rotation, and a fetal-like posture in the patient.

- *Planar inserts* are for patients with no deformity. (See Figure 6-12).
- *Curved/modular inserts* are for patients who require more contact of rounded surfaces.
- *Custom molded seat inserts* are for patients with severe fixed deformity (i.e., pelvis obliquity, windswept deformity). Custom molded seats distribute pressure well but transfer activities are difficult and weight-shifting ability is limited.[11]*

Local Shape

- *Split seat insert*—the front of the seat is cut back to accommodate a leg length discrepancy (Figure 7-5D).

---

* Also see Custom Molded Back Inserts.

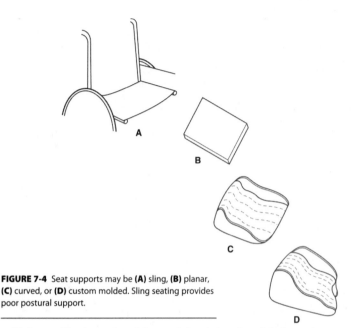

FIGURE 7-4 Seat supports may be **(A)** sling, **(B)** planar, **(C)** curved, or **(D)** custom molded. Sling seating provides poor postural support.

- *Undercut*—The front edge of the seat is beveled to clear tight hamstring tendons (Figure 7-5A).
- *Growth tail*—Additional seat material, hidden behind the back insert, can be used (moved forward) to increase seat depth as the patient grows (Figure 7-5C).

Advantages of Seat Inserts

- Offers support for patient's pelvis, hips, and thighs
- Can discourage a hammocking effect, which gives the patient a fetal-like appearance in the wheelchair.

Disadvantages of Seat Inserts

- Seat inserts and cushions raise the height of the seat resulting in potentially greater problems transferring, a higher center of gravity, a greater reach to the rear wheels for self-propulsion, and less knee clearance under tables (Figures 7-6A and B). Consider a hemi frame or hardware to lower the seat insert position to facilitate transfer. Consider an adjustable rear wheel axis to move the wheels up and closer to the hands to facilitate self-propulsion.
- Seat inserts add weight to the wheelchair.

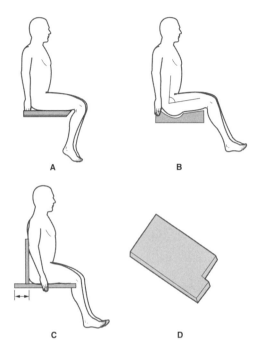

FIGURE 7-5 (A) Seat inserts can be tailored to the specific anthropomorphic needs of the patient. Seat inserts may be undercut or beveled on the front edge in patients with knee flexion contractures to provide additional clearance of tight hamstring tendons. **(B)** Antithrust seats help discourage forward sliding in the wheelchair for patients with adequate hip flexion. **(C)** Growth tails are extra seat material in the rear of the insert that can be used in the future to accommodate patient growth. **(D)** Split seats accommodate and support the thighs of patients with leg length discrepancies.

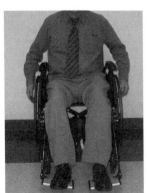

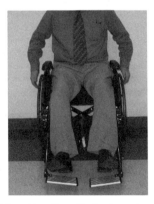

FIGURE 7-6 (A) Sitting without cushion. **(B)** Sitting with cushion will raise the user's position relative to the floor, underlying seat base, and handrims.

- Folding of the wheelchair is more difficult (i.e., insert must first be removed).
- Aggressively curved seat inserts (i.e., antithrust seats) may interfere with the patient's ability to transfer out of the wheelchair (Figure 7-5B).

Seat Height and Energy Cost of Propulsion

Van der Woude et al. reported a relationship between wheelchair seat height and the energy cost of propulsion (cardiopulmonary and kinematic performance) in a small, nonpatient sample ($n = 9$).[12] During propulsion in a treadmill protocol, oxygen costs increased 5% to 15%, mechanical efficiency diminished 0.5% to 1.0%, and the push range on the rim decreased 0.3 radians with increased seat height. (In other words, raising the user away from the handrims reduced mechanical efficiency and increased oxygen costs.) Based on cardiopulmonary responses, the authors recommended a seat height that would allow the user's hand to be directly on top of the handrim and the elbow angle to measure between 100 and 120 degrees, where full extension is defined as 180 degrees.

Inappropriate Seat Dimensions

The following are some of the problems found with incorrect seat dimensions (Figure 7-7):

- *If the seat is too deep*, the front of the seat may press into the back of the knees and cause the patient to slide forward in the wheelchair and sacral sit. *Based on my experience, excessive seat depth is one of the most common errors when fitting a wheelchair to a patient, and a frequent reason for sacral sitting.* In a case report of a man with C3–5 tetraplegia, his grade-2 ischial pressure ulcer failed to heal until the seat depth (along with back angle adjustments) was appropriately shortened.[13] Make sure excessive pressure does not exist between the front of the seat and back of the knee, causing patients to slide forward and sacral sit.
- *If the seat is too short*, the patient may not have enough support under their thighs and may slide forward. (Think of how unstable it is to sit on a bicycle seat.) There should be no more than a 2-inch gap between the back of the knee and the front edge of the seat once the patient is properly positioned to the rear of the seat.
- *If the seat is too wide*, the wheelchair may also be too wide. The patient may have difficulty reaching the rear wheels for self-propulsion[2] and may be at greater risk of developing scoliosis.[2] In general, seat width should be no more than 2 inches wider than the patient's hip-to-hip measurement.
- *If the seat is too high*, it may raise the patient too high off the floor, making transfers from the wheelchair difficult. Children and short adults need a low seat, whereas tall people require a higher seat.[2]
- *If the seat is too low*, the patient may be positioned too low at table surfaces.

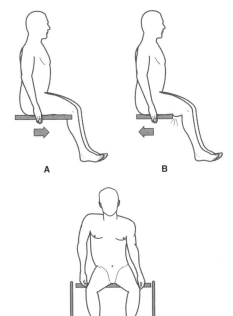

FIGURE 7-7 (A) If the seat insert is too deep, the front edge will press against the back of the knee, causing pressure and resulting in poor positioning with sacral sitting. Excessive seat depth is a very common error when fitting a wheelchair to a patient. **(B)** Short seat depth results in inadequate thigh support, excessive pressure under the distal posterior thigh, and the potential for forward sliding in the wheelchair. **(C)** A wide seat may result in difficulty self-propelling the wheelchair and inadequate postural support.

A   B

C

Comments

- The seat angle may be inclined 1 to 4 degrees above the horizon (front edge slightly higher than back edge) to help maintain the patient's position in the wheelchair.[8]
- "Squeezing the frame," that is, lowering the rear portion of the seat relative to the front portion while keeping the back insert angle unchanged, is thought to improve trunk stability, although there is a concern that it raises sitting pressure levels. In a *small, preliminary study* of seat inclination effects (squeezing) in 14-full time manual wheelchair users with complete paraplegia, Maurer and Sprigle found that changing inclination from 0 to 4 inches ($0°$ to $13.7°$) did not statistically alter peak pressures under the buttocks ($P = 0.60$) or *statistically* increase total force on seat.[14]* Contact area, however, decreased

* From 751.5 ± 184 N at $0°$ to 774.5 ± 187 N at $13.7°$; $P = 0.08$.

under the 13.7° compared to the 0° condition ($P = 0.03$). Although the findings of this small preliminary study are interesting (i.e., pressure under ischum may not necessarily increase with posterior seat inclination), interface pressures should be checked on an individual basis.

- *If the patient is a child*, make sure there is extra seat material toward the rear of the wheelchair (i.e., growth tail) that can be used as the patient grows.
- *If the patient has knee flexion contractures* or if the patient propels with the feet, make sure the front of the seat is beveled to allow for adequate clearance behind the knee.
- *If the patient tends to slide forward* but has full hip flexion range of motion, consider an antithrust seat. Sitting in an antithrust seat is a little like sitting in a bucket. The buttocks sink down into a trough and make it difficult to slide out. On the down side, transfers are more difficult and ischial pressure levels may be unacceptable (Figure 7-5B).

Seat Cushions

The main purposes of seat cushions are to provide comfort, support, and pressure reduction for the seated individual. It's important to understand that one cannot rely solely on a cushion to prevent pressure ulcer formation, nor will one type of cushion work for everyone.

During a seating evaluation, a variety of cushions should be evaluated so the best one for a particular patient can be selected. The cushion should provide pressure reduction under bony prominences, reduce pressure gradients, and maximize weight-bearing areas.[15] Other cushion considerations will be discussed below.

Wheelchair Cushion Classifications

There are several ways to classify cushions: by energy (static/passive vs. dynamic/battery-operated), material, shape, and coding procedures.

Material Classification

Static cushions,[16] that is, those not energized to do mechanical work, come in the form of solids, liquids, and gases and can generally be classified as being made from foam (Figure 7-8), gel/flotation (Figure 7-9), or air materials (Figure 7-10). Each technology has its advantages and disadvantages.[17]

Solid

Foam (Polyurethane)

- Lightweight
- Less expensive
- Poor heat conductor—can increase temperatures[18]
- Not moisture resistant[19]

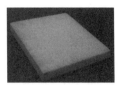

FIGURE 7-8 Foam cushions are lightweight and can be cut as needed, but have a limited shelf life.

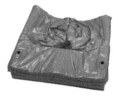

FIGURE 7-9 Gel cushion. (Courtesy of Sunrise Medical)

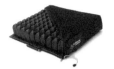

FIGURE 7-10 Air cushion. (Courtesy of The Roho Group)

- Wide variety to choose from[11]
- Cut to size
- Easy to transfer
- Stable base
- Readily available
- Breathable[11]
- Difficult to clean
- May wear out within 6 months
- Susceptible to pulling (tension), shear, and moisture[20]
- May lose support and pressure-relief properties[11]
- May not be the choice for a long-term user
- Deteriorates with sun exposure
- Deteriorates over time, even if not used[20]

Honeycomb Cushions
A relatively new type of solid cushion is composed of honeycomb-shaped units made of porous thermoplastic urethane. It is lightweight, cleanable, and provides air flow for cooler and dryer skin, as well as some shock absorption and postural support (Figure 7-11). Disadvantages include discomfort due to its firmness, and material compression, which can alter pressure distribution and require replacement.[17] Future studies may help to determine which types of individuals may benefit from these cushions.

Liquid (Flotation: Gel or Water)

Gel

- Gel or water/chemically filled
- Easy to clean
- Gel can be molded/positioned around/under bony prominences[19]
- Conducts heat away from skin[17]
- Gel is thought to simulate body fat[11]

- Adjusts to body movements[11]
- Heavy—an issue if propulsion efficiency is a priority or for car transfers if UEs are weak[20]
- Can leak
- Can develop consolidated hard localized area[20]
- Gel may need to be manually redistributed (kneaded)[19]
- User may develop intolerance for other cushion types[11]

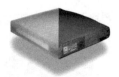

FIGURE 7-11 Honeycomb cushion. (Courtesy of Supracor)

Gas

Air-Filled

- Lightweight
- Easy to clean
- Compartmentalized
- Difficult to use in transfers (unstable)
- Unstable—may be critical issue in those with poor trunk control[16]
- Puncture prone (leak)
- Requires monitoring of pressure level

Combination of Above Materials (Hybrids)

Combine materials (gels, air, foam) in order to provide properties best suited for a particular patient.[11] For example, multiple layers of foam with different densities may be combined to achieve the desired level of support and comfort characteristics for a patient. Alternatively, fluid materials (gas/liquid) can address pressure issues while the solids (foams) can provide stability.[21]

Dynamic Seating (Alternating Therapy)

This type of seating offers a mechanical means for changing pressure areas under the user in the seat and requires an external power source (battery). Disadvantages may include added weight[11] and dependency on a power source.*

There is some limited evidence, at least in eight able-bodied volunteers, that skin tissue perfusion rates are higher and minimal interface seat pressure (MISP) values lower during dynamic cushion use (MISP 10.6 ± 7.6 mm Hg, while in its deflation cycle) as compared with a static gel (MISP 60.9 ± 10.5 mm Hg) and air cushion (MISP 69.1 ± 10.7 mm Hg), at least for the limited 20-minute data collection period in the study. Generalizability is limited, however, due to a nonpatient population.[22] Dynamic seating may serve a possible role if manual repositioning schedules are not adhered to consistently.

---

* Don't confuse dynamic seating as described above with a separate "dynamic" or "active" pediatric seating technology that permits a limited amount of hip and knee mobility while in the postural support system.

Shape Classification

Cushions also can be classified by shape. Planar, curved, and contoured cushions have been described earlier in this chapter in the seat inserts section.

Coding Classification

Medicare classifies seat cushions using codes to aid in product differentiation and reimbursement.[23] Four categories are recognized: general use, skin protection, positioning, and skin protection and positioning. Coding is determined by observing cushion behavior under standardized testing procedures. These tests include:

- *Immersion*—All cushions should permit a mechanical model to be immersed to a depth of 2.5 cm, but cushions in skin protection groups should immerse to 4 cm so the outside buttocks areas are involved in pressure distribution.
- *Interface pressures*—General use cushions may produce peak interface seating pressures under the ischium/sacrum/coccyx 25% greater than a reference cushion (i.e., 3 inches of thick flat foam). In contrast, skin protection cushion groups must show peak pressure values that are 15% less than the reference cushion.
- *Positioning capability*—Positioning cushions should have at least two features that offer structure to the cushion (e.g., lateral or medial thigh supports; areas of greater firmness within the cushion).
- *Lifespan*—Skin protection cushions should, through manufacturer testing, last longer under normal use (tested after 1½ years) compared to general use cushions (tested at 1 year).

Comments

- *No single best seat cushion exists for all patients.*[24]
- *No one cushion is best at preventing pressure ulcers.* Cullum et al.'s 2004 systematic review of three randomized clinical trials (RCTs) found that none of the cushions were better at preventing pressure ulcers.[25] Evidence was insufficient for an effect comparing gel with foam or foam with contoured foam cushions.
- Shopping for cushions involves multiple considerations including pressure-relieving properties, stability, ease in transfers, level of maintenance, and weight. Each patient should be individually evaluated with a variety of cushions.[11]
- Choose a cushion together with the wheelchair.[20,26] The fit of the patient will be affected by both the cushion and frame. Evaluate and order both at the same time whenever possible.
- As noted in the seat inserts section, cushions raise the individual from the seat and wheels, affecting handrim reach and knee clearance under tables.
- Covers keep cushions clean (consider getting more than one for laundering). Covers can affect moisture, temperatures, and air exchange at the seat interface, but just as important, can alter the shape and pressure distribution of the cushion if the cover is ill fitting or does not stretch.[19,20] Try to use cushion

covers and cushions that allow for air exchange so that moisture and heat buildup does not occur between the skin and cushion—both are risk factors for ulcer formation.[20]

- Periodically inspect cushions (with their cover off) to determine if (1) cushion material is fatigued and needs replacement, and (2) the cushion is correctly oriented and installed in the wheelchair (i.e., targeting the ischia).[23] Signs of cushion fatigue include fissures, cracks, or compression in foam cushions; material cracks leading to leaks in air cushions; or gel/liquid oozing and alterations in gel consistency (areas of firmness and softness) in gel cushions.[23]
- If the patient is not at risk for skin breakdown, *foam* material (solid) may be sufficient for comfort. If the patient is at risk for skin breakdown, *cushions* need to be evaluated to determine the best pressure-reducing cushion for that particular patient. Pressure mapping devices may be helpful in selecting a cushion for a particular patient if the device is reliable and valid (see Chapter 3, Clinical Examination).
- *Avoid donut-type cushions* because they may cause venous congestion and predispose the patient to pressure ulcers.[27]

Lateral Trunk Supports

Lateral trunk supports (lateral thoracic supports[1]) are side support structures for the patient's torso (Figure 7-12).

Purpose

- Provides lateral support and alignment for the trunk
- Acts as a tactile reminder to sit upright

Indications

- Patients with poor or fair trunk balance and control
- Patients who fall to the side[28]
- Patients with scoliosis.[28] For neuromuscular scoliosis in nonambulatory persons with cerebral palsy (CP), a three-point force configuration of thoracic/pelvic supports has been shown to have immediate effects (see Chapter 3, Clinical Examination, on Postural Alignment).[29]

Disadvantages

- Brachial plexus injuries may occur if lateral supports press into axilla.
- Reduced space for thick (e.g., winter) clothing.
- Positioning may restrict arm movements (e.g., propulsion, reaching).
- Patient may rely on thoracic support rather than using their own muscles to sit upright.
- Adds weight to wheelchair.

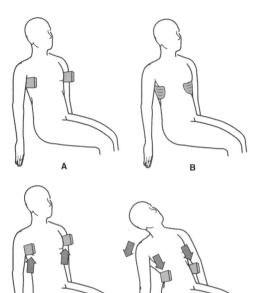

FIGURE 7-12 (A) Planar lateral supports provide trunk support in the coronal plane. **(B)** Contoured lateral supports offer greater pressure distribution. **(C)** Lateral trunk supports that press into the axilla can cause neurovascular problems. **(D)** Lateral trunk supports that are too low offer inadequate coronal support.

Types

Lateral trunk supports may be *planar* or *contoured* (curved) around the sides of the trunk.

- *Planar*—Provide flat padded support
- *Contoured (curved)*—Provide more contact and pressure distribution over the rounded trunk surfaces but may make it more difficult for patients to transfer out of the wheelchair because the supports curve around the side of the trunk (see Figure 6-13)
- *Swing-away hardware*—Allow lateral trunk supports to swing out of the way to facilitate transfers or while reclined in a wheelchair

Comments

- *If using a reclining frame*, seriously consider using *swing-away lateral trunk supports* so the lateral supports do not ride up into the axilla of the patient as the back is reclined.

- *If the lateral trunk supports are positioned too far apart* so they do not physically contact the sides of the patient, they may not function effectively to support the trunk in an upright position.
- *If the lateral trunk supports are positioned too close together,* less than the patient's chest width, they could cause excessive pressure into the sides of the chest, interfering with breathing and trunk movements, and causing pressure ulcers.
- *If the lateral trunk supports are positioned too high into the axilla,* they could cause excessive pressure, circulatory compromise, and nerve injuries to the brachial plexus.
- *If the lateral trunk supports are positioned too low,* below the costal level, they may not function effectively to support the trunk in midline.
- *If the lateral trunk supports are too thick,* they may interfere with arm movements. Consider making the laterals as thin as possible, 1 inch in thickness or less.
- *Gravity-assisted backward tilt* may improve tolerance for lateral supports in patients with scoliosis.[4]

Anterior Trunk Supports

These provide support for the front of the patient's chest area and/or over each shoulder (Figure 7-13).[1] The patient with poor sitting balance, weak trunk musculature, and whose trunk lists forward, may need anterior trunk support.

Advantages

- Prevents the trunk and shoulders from falling forward[4]
- May assist in keeping the shoulders from protracting
- May provide stability if shoulders elevate[4]

Disadvantages

- Safety issue of strangulation—if the patient slides forward the chest harness could ride up to the neck area.[30,31]
- If support is too tightly secured over the chest, it may interfere with reaching and breathing.

Types of Anterior Trunk Supports

There are many chest harness styles, although their unique advantages are not always striking. In my opinion, a chest harness may be useful in keeping the trunk from falling completely forward but may not markedly improve postural alignment. Consider gravity-assisted positioning using tilt or reclining frames to minimize reliance on trunk supports, improve trunk alignment, and reduce the risk of chest harness–related injuries.

Chest harnesses are available in the following types:

- *H chest harness*—Is shaped like the letter "H"
- *Butterfly harness*—Is shaped like a butterfly

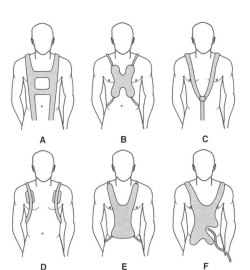

FIGURE 7-13 Anterior trunk supports: **(A)** H harness, **(B)** butterfly harness, **(C)** V harness, **(D)** shoulder harness, **(E)** vest harness, **(F)** custom harness, **(G)** chest strap, **(H)** shoulder retractors. **(I)** Strangulation can occur if a chest harness if improperly donned or the patient slides forward in the wheelchair.

- *V chest harness*—Is shaped like a letter "V." Straps provide greater clearance under the neck but they may cut into the sides of the patient's neck if not padded.
- *Vest harness*—Provides maximal contact with the trunk
- *Custom harness*—Traced to the shape of the patient with deformity or special needs
- *Shoulder harness*—Provides a posterior force for each shoulder like a backpack but may interfere with forward reaching ability

In addition,

- **Shoulder retractors** are padded rigid supports that hook over each shoulder to help retract the shoulders and help prevent the trunk from listing forward. These devices severely restrict trunk mobility, could interfere with UE mobility, and may not be tolerated by all patients.

- **Chest belts (straps)** are straps secured across the patient's chest rather than over the shoulders, as is the case with a chest harness, and may offer gentle support to sit upright.[4] Chest belts interfere less with upper extremity movements but are not as effective in keeping shoulders back.

Comments

- In the clinic, you may observe chest belts used more in persons with adult spinal cord injury (SCI) tetraplegia and chest harnesses used more in children with CP.
- Make sure the chest harness provides good clearance of the neck to avoid strangulation.[31]
- Make sure the chest harness does not press against or occlude gastrointestinal tubes or other lines exiting the patient's abdominal/chest wall.
- Make sure the patient's shoulders are sufficiently broad on each side so the shoulder strap portion of the harness can drape over the shoulder. Some patients are endowed with a very narrow area between the neck and shoulder, thus offering a small purchase area for the strap to drape over. In this case, consider a *chest belt*.
- The harness should not be secured using the seat (pelvic) belt. Instead, use four separate straps for the harness.
- Donning the harness: The bottom two straps of the harness should be secured and tightened before the top two straps are adjusted in order to avoid having the harness ride up into the patient's neck area.

Armrests

Armrests (arm supports[1]) are support structures for the arms, located on each side of the mobility base.[9]

Advantages

- Support upper extremities[2]
- Assist in weight shifting and pressure reduction[2]
- Support during transfers
- Protect clothes from elements/dirt if side panels included[8]

Armrests and Body Weight

Armrests may support some of the body weight of individuals with SCI while sitting in a wheelchair. In Gilsdorf et al.'s study, armrests supported about 9% and 5% of the body weight of persons with paraplegia ($n = 6$) and tetraplegia ($n = 5$), respectively.[32] This makes sense because UEs have mass and they would contribute to the patient's total body mass if not for their support by armrests. Their finding, however, failed to reach a statistical significance at a conventional 0.05 level, perhaps due to low power (i.e., small sample size).

Types of Armrest Features

The following are some of the available armrest features[24,26] (Figure 7-14):

- *No armrests*—Patient has no UE support but good access to wheels for propulsion and sliding board/side transfers (see Figure 6-11).
- *Fixed*—Nonremovable, durable, and lighter weight[33] (see Figure 6-8)
- *Swing away/swing back*—Moves armrests to the rear to facilitate transfers.
- *Removable*—Facilitates sliding board and two-person assisted transfer lifts to and from wheelchair. Removable armrests add width to wheelchair (about 2 inches).[2]
- *Full-length*—Assists UEs in transfers, provides support for patients with lordoses and obesity,[2] and supports lap board use. Access to desk areas will be limited (see Figure 6-8).
- *Desk-length*—Provides access to a work surface but may offer only partial UE support (see Figure 6-6).

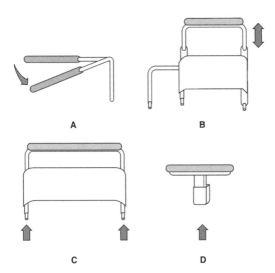

A **B**

C **D**

FIGURE 7-14 Types of armrest features: **(A)** Tubular arms may swing away and allow greater access to handrims. **(B)** Desk-length armrests enable closer access under tables. Adjustable height armrests enable up or down arm pad positioning to properly support the UEs and facilitate pressure relief weight shifts as well as UE push-off during transfers. **(C)** Full-length armrests provide greater length to facilitate push-off during stand pivot transfers and offers a supportive surface for a lap board. Double-posted armrests provide a durable base for patients who are rough on equipment. **(D)** Armrests with single posting allows easier removal of armrests.

- *Tubular, padded*—Not strong but greater access to rear wheels[3]
- *Adjustable height*—To optimize amount of UE support; adjust height of armrests during transfers; adjust lap tray height; adjust height as children grow.[3]
- *Double posted*—Stronger than single-post arms but more difficult to remove.
- *Single posted*—Provides UE support, easy to remove, but not durable.
- *Double length*—Provides sideways protection for reclining frames.[3] Longer lengths may also be available.
- *Wraparound*—Reduces frame width.[10]

Comments

If Armrests Are Too Low

- Poor posture (slumped)
- Increased fatigue
- Respiration can be affected

If Armrests Are Too High

- Elevated scapula
- Interfere with handrim reach for self-propulsion

Clothes Guard

The clothes guard (skirt guard) is located on the sides of the wheelchair seat near the armrests to protect the user from wheel debris.[24]

Lap Board

A lap board (lap tray; upper extremity support surface[3]) is a rigid flat board secured over the armrests that functions as a table surface (Figure 1-1).[1] Lap boards provide a surface for eating, school work, communication devices, and UE support while the patient is in the wheelchair. The lap board may interfere with independent transfer ability.

Advantages

- Work area on the wheelchair instead of using a desk[2,34]
- Support surface for feeding[34]
- Surface for communication boards[34]
- May provide a surface to mount sensors for power wheelchair controls[35]
- Provides a weight-bearing surface for the UEs to assist in upper body support
- Protects arm from falling for patients with sensory neglect[36]
- Increases awareness of an arm for patients with sensory neglect[36]

Disadvantages

- Lap boards may interfere with the patient's ability to propel the wheelchair, reach for wheel locks, and transfer out of the wheelchair. Consider having the sides of the board narrowed near the wheels to improve reach for the wheels.
- Adds weight to the wheelchair. (This is no small matter. I've been accosted in the street by a mother who complained about the excess weight of her daughter's board.)
- May interfere with visual and tactile exploration of body parts.
- If there is a history of injury due to limbs or head hitting the board surface, consider padding the surface causing injury (i.e., pad top of board for head and upper limbs; under board for knees banging). The board can also cause pressure to the trunk if the patient slides forward into it. Address the problem of sliding by stabilizing the pelvis. If the problem persists, consider padding the inner rim of the board to protect the trunk.
- A lap board may act as a restraint if the patient cannot independently remove it.
- Based on a 2008 systematic review, evidence is insufficient to support the use of a lap board for shoulder subluxation prevention in persons poststroke.[37]

Comments

- *Lap boards are either solid (nonclear) or clear.* Consider a clear board for patients with adequate vision so they can view their lower limbs through the tray.
- *If the patient will perform upper limb skills,* make sure the armrests are adjustable in height so the lap board can be optimally positioned for UE activities.
- *If the patient flexes lower limb*s and hits knees into the bottom of the board, consider padding the board bottom.
- *If the board is too low,* it may not provide enough support for the upper limbs. In addition, it may force the patient to strain in order to view objects at the lower visual level.
- *If the board is too high,* it may force the patient's shoulders up toward the ears (scapula elevation). Consider a board height from the seat equal to the distance from the top of the seat cushion to the elbow (with the arm vertically aligned) plus 1 inch.[38]
- *If there is too much of a gap* between the abdomen and the inside of the board, the patient's arm may get caught between the board and their trunk. In addition, food or other objects may fall through this gap if it is too wide. Although needs may vary, consider about a 1-inch gap between the abdomen and the inside of the board.
- *If there is not enough gap* between the abdomen and the inside of the board, the patient may not have enough space for winter coats, weight changes, and breathing.
- The lap board must be removed and stored securely during school bus transportation so it does not become a projectile during a sudden stop.[39]

FIGURE 7-15
Protraction blocks can encourage midline positioning of the UEs.

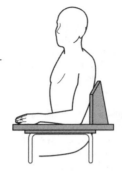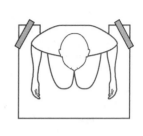

Protraction Blocks

Protraction blocks (shoulder protraction wings,[4] humeral blocks[3]) are rigid pads mounted posterior-laterally on the lap board or the back of the frame (Figure 7-15).

Advantages

- Encourages midline posture on the UEs[4]
- May prevent shoulders from extending and falling behind the wheelchair
- May prevent excessive scapula retraction by blocking associated horizontal abduction at the shoulder

Comments

- Protraction blocks are very useful on backward tilt-in-space wheelchairs because gravity will tend to pull the patient's UEs into extension as the frame tilts backward.
- UEs may lift over the protraction block, defeating the purpose of the part.
- The clinician may have to experiment with the placement of the protraction blocks before determining the best position for a particular patient.
- Adds weight to the wheelchair.

Hip Guides

Hip guides (hip blocks) are a support structure located on the sides of the seat near the hips (Figure 7-16). They help center the patient's pelvis toward the center of the seat to encourage midline posture while sitting.

Advantages

- Guides the hips and pelvis toward the center of the seat
- Encourages midline positioning of the upper body

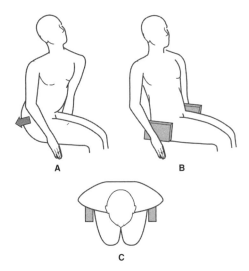

FIGURE 7-16
(A) Patient with pelvis deviated out of midline without hip guides. **(B)** Patient using hip guides with pelvis centered and trunk in midline. **(C)** Patient with hip guides (aerial view).

Disadvantages

- Increases the weight of the wheelchair
- Decreases the useable width of the seat because it takes up space

Comments

- If hip guides are positioned too close together, less than the hip-to-hip width of the patient, pressure ulcers can develop at the hips (greater trochanters). Transfers into a wheelchair may also be more difficult.
- If hip guides are positioned too far apart (e.g., greater than about an inch from each hip), they may not function to guide the pelvis to the center of the seat, causing the patient to sit asymmetrically.

Knee Adductors

Knee adductors (lateral thigh supports[1]) are support structures located on the sides of the seat near the knees (Figure 7-17) and are useful for patients who sit with excessive hip abduction.

Advantage

- Prevents hips from abducting excessively

FIGURE 7-17
(A) Patient with excessive hip abduction (i.e.,"frog" position of LEs). **(B)** Knee adductors prevent excessive hip abduction of the LEs. **(C)** Patient with knee adductors (aerial view).

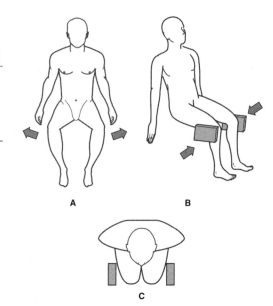

Disadvantage

• Adds weight to the wheelchair

Comments

• Make sure the knee adductor will not cause excessive pressure over the peroneal nerve near the fibula head.
• *If the knee adductors are positioned too close together*, so that the knees are pressed together, it may be more difficult to transfer into the wheelchair. In addition, it may promote adductor contractures and poor hip joint development. Finally, knee adduction is contraindicated in patients following hip arthroplasty surgery.
• *If the knee adductors are positioned too far apart* and do not touch the lateral knee, they may not function to block undesirable hip abduction and hence may promote contractures of the hip abductors and external rotators.

Anterior Knee Blocks

Anterior knee blocks are padded structures in front of each knee that prevent anterior displacement of the knees and therefore indirectly prevent forward pelvic sliding.

Comments

- Interferes with transfers.
- Deleterious effects if forces acting through the knees are excessive or if hip/femoral pathology exists.
- Soft tissue inflammation may result from repetitive rubbing of knees against knee blocks.

Pommels

A pommel (medial leg separator, medial thigh separator;[1] medial knee block[3]) is a padded structure located between the knees (Figure 7-18). The pommel helps promote normal hip development and minimize the possibility of adduction contractures.

Advantages

- Prevents hip adductor contractures by keeping knees apart
- Prevents knees from pressing together, which can result in pressure ulcers
- Maintains hip joints in an abducted position for normal development and reduces the possibility of hip subluxation or dislocation[4]

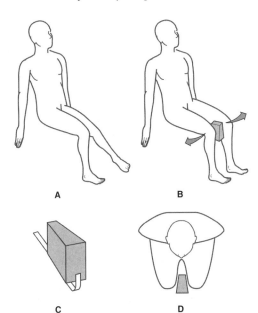

FIGURE 7-18 (A) Patient without pommel exhibits an LE scissoring posture. **(B)** Patient with pommel maintains hip abduction and knees apart. **(C)** Pommel with hardware. **(D)** Patient with pommel (aerial view).

A   B

C   D

Disadvantages

- Interferes with transfers; consider a removable pommel
- Groin pressure and discomfort may occur if patient slides forward into pommel.
- Adds weight to the wheelchair.
- Hardware (metal) from the pommel can result in injuries if the patient kicks or presses into it. (In these cases, try to "hide" hardware under the seat or pad hardware.)

Comments

- *Keep pommel distal.* Pommels should not be located near the patient's groin area. Proximal placement may stimulate the hip adductors.[4]
- Pommels should not be used to prevent sliding out of wheelchairs because groin injuries can result.
- *If pommel is positioned too far posteriorly* in the seat, groin pressure can result.
- *If pommel is positioned too far anteriorly* in the seat, it may be located in front of the patient's knees and therefore not function to keep the knees apart.
- *If pommel is too wide*, the patient who is flexible may be forced into excessive hip abduction.
- *If the patient has tight knee adductors*, then a wide pommel may cause pressure ulceration over the medial condyles of the knees.

Wheel Locks

Wheel locks (brakes, parking locks[2]) are metal devices on each side of the wheelchair that press into the rear tires (Figure 7-19).[40]

Advantages

- Locks the rear wheels to prevent the wheelchair from moving once parked
- Provides stability during transfers[5]

Types

Toggle, level,[2] and scissor are three types of wheel lock designs found on most wheelchairs.

Toggle

The toggle design requires the user to apply anterior or posterior forces to engage the wheel lock. The amount of compression of the lock against the tire is preset (see Figure 6-6 and Figure 7-20).[3]

Toggle type wheel locks come in two configurations (push to lock and pull to lock) depending on which direction you wish to lock them in. If the patient can

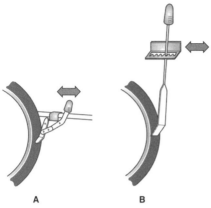

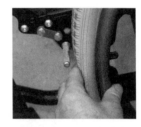

FIGURE 7-19 (left) **(A)** Toggle wheel locks have a preset tension and require a pulling or pushing force. **(B)** Level wheel locks have variable set tension against the tires and require some medial/lateral manipulation to operate. **(C)** A brake extension facilitates reach and gives the patient a mechanical advantage to engage the wheel lock.

A   B

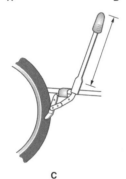

FIGURE 7-20 (above) Toggle brake (with low air pressure in adjacent tire).

C

self-propel the wheelchair, consider pull-to-lock wheel locks so the wheel locks are not accidentally engaged as the patient propels the wheels forward.

Level

The level design requires coordination[3] and some medial/lateral manipulation by the user in order to engage the lock into notches. The amount of compression of the lock against the tire (and therefore the "holding power") varies and depends on which notch is selected[3] (see Figure 7-19B).

Scissor

Located beneath the seat, these wheel locks are less likely to catch on clothing (see Figure 6-11).[6]

Location on Frame

- *High mount*—Easier to reach but may interfere with propulsion[24]
- *Low mount*—Requires better hand function, is harder to reach, but will not interfere with propulsion and there is a reduced risk of injuries to fingers during rapid propulsion[26]

Attendant-Operated Wheel Locks

These locks allow easy access for the attendant (i.e., attached toward the rear of the wheelchair), but not easy access for the patient.

Grade Aids/Hill Climbers

These facilitate forward propulsion uphill to maintain forward momentum; prevent backward rolling.[10]

Comments

- *Wheel locks must be engaged for safety whenever the patient transfers into or out of the wheelchair.* Patients can potentially sustain serious injuries (i.e., hip fractures or worse) during transfers if the wheelchair rolls away from them.
- The wheelchair may still move (slide) if the wheel locks are engaged but the floor is waxed (low friction) or the pneumatic rear tires have low pressure (Figure 7-20). Maintain recommended air pressures in tires.
- The bus driver must secure the frame of the wheelchair to the floor of the bus for safety (tie-down system). Otherwise, the entire wheelchair (even with wheel locks engaged) would move if the bus stopped abruptly.
- If the patient has difficulty reaching or engaging the wheel locks, consider installing a *brake extension*, which is a long metal tube that attaches to the brake handle (see next section).

Brake Extension

A brake extension is a 6- to 9-inch extended removable metal arm that facilitates reach and engagement of wheel locks (see Figure 6-2). Brake extensions make reach easier and provide a mechanical advantage to engage wheel locks. In a study of the frequency of wheelchair mobility in nursing homes, Simmons et al. found one reason for nonuse was the inability of residents to disengage the wheel locks on their wheelchair so they could propel. (Locks were stuck or rusted.) Brake extensions may have been useful in fostering independence in this case.[41]

Comments

- The long lever length of the brake extension can cause excessive torque that can result in damage to the brake.
- Because brake extensions are located near the rear wheels and extend into the air, they may interfere with manual propulsion and transfer activities.[3]
- Brake extensions can potentially be used as weapons by aggressive patients because they are removable. Some extensions can be ordered with a chain for attachment to the wheelchair.

Rear Wheels

The rear wheels enable the wheelchair to roll (Figure 7-21).[24]

Type

Spoke (see also Figure 6-2)

- Lighter weight[10]
- Requires maintenance

Molded (Spokeless, Mag) (see also Figure 6-6)

- Heavier[3]
- Low maintenance[2]
- More durable[10]

Size

Rear wheels range from 20 to 26 inches in diameter. As diameter increases, turning radius increases and maneuvering becomes more difficult.

- Standard size = 24-inch diameter

- Hemiplegic chairs have 22-inch diameter wheels.

FIGURE 7-21
(A) Spoke wheels are lightweight but require maintenance. **(B)** Molded (spokeless) wheels require low maintenance and are durable, but are heavier than spoke wheels.

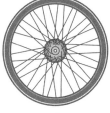

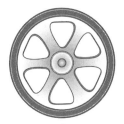

A   B

Camber (Wheel Angle)

Cambered rear wheels are angled so the top of the wheel is tilted medially while the bottom of the wheel is tilted out laterally (see Figure 6-3).[24] Cambered rear wheels improve the patient's lateral stability and ease in steering the wheelchair[10,26] but increase the width of the wheelchair, potentially limiting access through doorways. Camber can also reduce backward stability. Using Canadian database records ($n = 374$), Trudel et al. found an almost four-fold increased risk of instability with camber usage.[42] A statistically significant percentage of instability incidences were in the backward direction.

Advantages

- Easier to steer[26]
- Improves reach to handrims (ergonomics)[43]
- Increases lateral stability
- Increases turning stability[26]
- Less tendency for downward turning on slopes[43]
- Protects hands when going through doorways[43]

Disadvantages

- Increases width of wheelchair—difficulty clearing doorways[26]
- Reduces rearward stability
- Decreases wheelchair height[43]
- Increases or has no effect on energy cost of propulsion (controversial)[43]

Rear Tires

Rear tires provide a rolling surface, traction, and shock absorption for rear wheels.[24,26] The three major categories are *pneumatic (air filled)*,[44] *solid rubber tires*, and *airless (filled)*.

Pneumatic

- Good shock absorption
- Comfortable ride[2]
- Lower rolling resistance[33]
- Prolongs life of wheelchair[2]
- Lighter weight
- Use on carpet, gravel, and grass
- Good for outdoor use[10]
- Good on uneven ground[10]
- Maintenance problems (punctures).[3] Consider purchasing an air pump.[3]

Tire Pressure and Rolling Resistance

To make propulsion easier, maintain correct tire pressure. Low tire pressure (pneumatics) increases rolling resistance and can lead to greater energy expenditure. Sawatzky and Denison reported a 15% increase in energy expenditure as measured by heart rate in 10 children and adolescents with spina bifida (T6 or lower) when propelling wheelchairs with a reduced tire pressure rating of 25 psi.[45]

In adults with paraplegia (*n* = 15; level T5–12), Sawatzky et al. found a 12% significant increase in energy expenditure (O_2, heart rate measures) with tires inflated to 50% of recommended levels.[46] Even so, pneumatic tires fared better than solid rubber tires. During rolling resistance testing, pneumatic tires traveled greater distances than solid tires, even when pneumatics were markedly underinflated (25%). Check tire pressure periodically because 50% pressure loss can occur within a month's time.

Solid Rubber Tires

- Indoor use[2]
- Durable[3]
- No maintenance problems
- Less shock absorption
- Use on smooth surfaces[2]
- Good on hard floors (e.g., nursing home)[10]

Airless (Solid Insert; Flat-Free Inserts)

- No maintenance problems[24]
- Shock absorption better than solid rubber but not as good as pneumatics

Tread Surface on Tire

- Improves traction[10]
- Use on soft, sandy, and rough terrain[2]

Adjustable Rear Axle

Adjustable rear axle hardware allows the rear wheel to be optimally repositioned relative to the user's UE in a wheelchair to make propulsion easier (Figure 7-22). *Whenever possible, handrim wheelchair users (especially persons with paraplegia) should have adjustable axle hardware included on their order (also see Chapter 4 Functional Examination).* Although axle adjustability is typically included on ultralight wheelchairs, the feature may be limited or absent on depot-style and lightweight frames.

FIGURE 7-22 An adjustable rear axle can allow rear wheels to be positioned forward to optimize the user's propulsion efficiency.

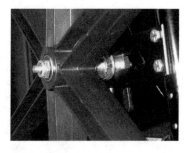

Rear Axle Adjustability and Pushrim Biomechanics

Moving the rear wheel axle anteriorly can improve propulsion biomechanics. In an observational study involving 40 persons with paraplegia (traumatic SCI at least 1 year postinjury), Boninger et al. found fair to moderate partial correlation coefficients (associations = 0.34 to 0.46) between rear axle position and pushrim biomechanic variables.[47] As the axle position moved forward (anteriorly), push angle increased, propulsion frequency decreased, and force rise rates diminished. These outcomes are desirable because they reduce potentially high reactive forces within the shoulder as users contact the pushrim and also reduce how often the user needs to exert force on the rim to travel. Adjustable rear axles are an important method for attempting to minimize UE stresses associated with overuse injuries in manual wheelchair users.

Handrims

Handrims are circular tubes attached to the rear wheels (see Figure 6-2).

Advantages

- Provide a grip surface for self-propulsion
- Control soiling of hands

Size

The size of handrims acts in a similar way to the gears on a bicycle and provide either a speed or power advantage.[10]

Small Diameter Rims

If small diameter rims are used (i.e., 12- or 15-inch), the seat may need to be lowered and the wheels cambered to aid reach.[33]

- Speed advantage[10] (good for sports)
- Easier to maintain speed[26]

Large Diameter Rims

- Power advantage[10] (good if weak)
- Starts and acceleration are easier[26]

Types of Handrims

- *Standard*—Uncoated rims
- *Vinyl/plastic/foam coated*—Provides firm, comfortable grip on handrims for self-propulsion.[3,26] Foam increases friction to facilitate propulsion.[6] Finger burns due to the increased friction coefficient of the handrim coating can result.[26]
- *Projections*—To assist propulsion if difficulty gripping or hand deformity. The spacing,[10] orientation (straight or oblique),[10] and shape (knobs)[3] of the projections may vary.
- *Flexible handrims*—High friction elastic handrims are designed to conform to the hand, improve comfort and grip, and may result in less muscle activity to grip. Richter et al. found that 25 wheelchair users (most with SCI below T5) required less wrist and finger flexor electromyography (EMG) activity using flexible handrims compared to standard uncoated ones while being tested on a research treadmill.[48]

Spokeguard

A spokeguard is a covering over the outer spokes of each wheel used to protect the fingers.[24]

Casters

Casters are small wheels, usually in the front, that enable the wheelchair to turn and steer (Figure 7-23).[24] From an engineering perspective, casters are probably the first line of defense during impacts with obstacles such as curbs and cracks.

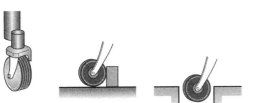

FIGURE 7-23 (A) Casters enable the wheelchair to turn and steer. **(B)** Small casters do not roll over obstacles well and can get caught in cracks.

A   B

Size

Casters range in size from 2 to 8 inches in diameter.

Larger (see Figure 6-6)

- Better shock absorption (better ride) but less maneuverability
- Rolls easier over obstacles[26]
- Lowers rolling resistance[49]
- Performs well outdoors[33]

Smaller (see Figure 6-3)

- Smaller turning radius for easier and quicker turning (good for sports)[10,26]
- Minimal flutter[26]
- Clears front rigging (footplates) better than larger casters
- More easily get caught in potholes and sidewalk cracks[3]
- Less shock absorption (rough ride)[26]
- Performs well indoors except for carpet[33]

Wider (Ball Shaped)

- Improves rolling resistance and use on sand[49]

Pin Locks

Pin locks help to stabilize the casters during transfers.[3]

Caster Tires

Caster tires provide a rolling surface, traction, and shock absorption for casters.[24]

Pneumatics

- Good shock absorption
- May improve durability and life cycle cost of wheelchair[50]
- Comfortable ride[3]
- Lightweight[3]
- Maintenance problems (i.e., punctures)[3]
- Can use outdoors[2,26,44]

Solid Tires

- No maintenance problems

- Less shock absorption; less comfortable ride
- Use indoors[2]

Semipneumatics

- Comfortable ride
- Puncture-proof but heavier and more difficult to propel[3]
- Can use outdoors[2]

Caster Tires and Life Cycle Costs

One interesting finding that emerged from Cooper et al.'s study of life cycle costs of wheelchairs is that the rehabilitation wheelchairs tested with 8-inch *pneumatic casters* ($n = 3$) did far better on fatigue tests and lasted three times longer than the same chair models tested using 8-inch solid casters ($n = 6$).[50] In other words, upgrading to pneumatic caster tires may extend the life of a chair markedly.

Seat Belts

A seat belt (positioning belt,[3] pelvic belt[1]) is a strap on the seat that is secured across the patient's hips.

Advantages

- Used as a positioning belt[3] to maintain proper body alignment and pelvic position
- Prevents forward sliding in the wheelchair
- Prevents LE extensor thrust[26]

Types

Choose a fastener that can be easily operated by the patient (Figure 7-24).

- *Velcro*—Requires grasp and pulling to open the belt. Velcro may be too weak for use as a seat belt, particularly because it wears out with use.
- *Buckle*—Requires grasp and pull to open belt.
- *Fastex (plastic that opens when the sides are squeezed)*—Requires opposition of thumb and digits to open belt.
- *Auto (push the button to open)*—May require finger action, wrist flexion, or shoulder internal rotation to open belt.
- *Airplane (lift the handle to open)*—May require wrist extension or shoulder external rotation to open belt.

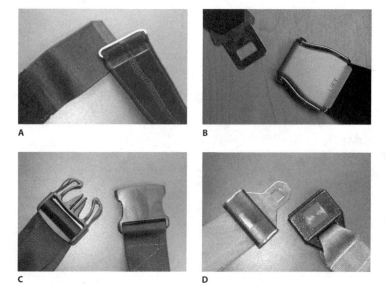

FIGURE 7-24 Seat belt styles: **(A)** Velcro, **(B)** airplane, **(C)** Fastex, **(D)** auto belt.

Size

Seat belts are sized to accommodate a range of body types:

- *Small children*—1 inch wide[3]
- *Large children*—1.5 inches wide[3]
- *Adults*—2 inches wide[3]
- *Large/obese adults*—Extra long

Orientation of Seat Belts and Other Pelvic Positioning Devices

The seat belt can be oriented to achieve different seating goals (Figure 7-25).

- *45 degrees*—Usually effective in maintaining pelvic positioning
- *90 degrees*—Less restrictive; enables pelvis to anteriorly tilt[3]
- *Peroneal straps*—Additional straps (wraps around each thigh, usually in a medial to lateral direction); may help discourage forward sliding of the pelvis. Avoid compression of sensitive structures such as the femoral artery.[3]
- *Attendant-operated belt*—Provides convenient belt access for the caregiver when the patient cannot operate the seat belt

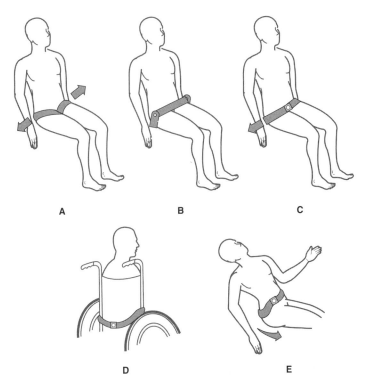

FIGURE 7-25 (A) Peroneal straps, secured across each thigh, may help discourage forward sliding of the pelvis. **(B)** The sub-ASIS bar is an aggressive approach to maintaining pelvic positioning in a patient who exhibits very strong extensor activity and forward sliding behavior. **(C)** Many patients generally do well with only a seat belt oriented at a 45-degree angle. **(D)** Attendant-operated belt location offers easy access for the caregiver when the patient cannot operate the seat belt. **(E)** If seat belt is positioned across the waist instead of the hips, forward sliding may occur.

Disadvantage

- Seat belts may act as a restraint if the patient cannot independently operate the belt. Try to order a buckle that the patient can open or close independently. Also, have the buckle installed in a location where the patient can reach. Buckles positioned near the greater trochanters may be too difficult for the patient to operate.

Comments

- The seat belt is typically attached to the frame of the wheelchair with the belt angled 45 degrees up from the seat to maintain a midline pelvis.[4] Another option is to secure the seat belt at a 90-degree angle.
- *If the seat belt is too high* (i.e., at the level of the umbilicus) the patient may be able to "do the limbo" and slide underneath the seat belt. Make sure the seat belt is positioned *across the hips* and not the waist. If the buckle is at the level of the umbilicus, it's too high (see Figure 7-25E).
- *If the patient has a bony pelvis*, consider placing a pressure-relieving pad between the buckle and the patient.
- *If the seat belt is too loose*, the patient could slide forward until he or she makes contact with the belt. *This is probably the most common reason why patients slide*. As a rough guide, tighten seat belts so that you can fit only two fingers between the belt and the patient's abdomen.

Sub-ASIS Bar

The sub-ASIS bar (anterior superior iliac spine, pelvic stabilizer) is a rigid pelvic restraint (i.e., a round, padded, metal bar) positioned below the patient's ASIS (Figure 7-25B).[28]

Indication

- To prevent strong extensor thrusting out of the wheelchair

Disadvantages

- May be difficult for caregiver to install and remove the bar
- Interferes with independent transfers

Comments

- Some patients with severe extensor activity may actually bend the metal bar.
- May be difficult to properly position the bar.
- Monitor the patient's skin for pressure ulcers on the anterior pelvis.

Front Rigging*

Front rigging refers to both the footrest and the leg rest.[2] It provides a support surface for the feet and consists of a support bracket and footplate (Figure 7-26).[40] *The front rigging is vulnerable to impact loads from the LE (extensor spasticity) as well as the environment (curbs, door thresholds).*[33]

---

* Numerous, often ill-defined terms have been used in the literature to describe LE supports, including *hangers, brackets, leg rests*, and *foot supports*.

Indications

- Prevents feet from dragging on floor during transportation[2]
- Supports the distal thigh from pressure at the front edge of the seat so restricted circulation in that region is prevented[2]
- Places the knee joint in the required angle of knee extension or flexion
- Supports the ankle joint in the required amount of dorsiflexion
- May improve user stability in the chair (based on tests using test dummies)[51]

Types of Front Rigging

- *Fixed front rigging with flip-up footplates*—Durable; enables access for transfers but does not swing away for use in tight quarters[24]
- *Swing-away*—Better access for transfers but less durable and increased weight[26]
- *Detachable*—For maneuvering into small spaces (e.g., bathrooms)[2,26]
- *Elevating leg rests*—Support both leg and foot at multiple knee angle positions and may be indicated for casted legs, arthrodesed knees, and orthostatic hypotension (see Figure 6-6).[24]* Elevating leg rests, however, increase both the weight and overall length of the wheelchair and are contraindicated if the patient presents with hamstring tightness.[3] Finally, contrary to popular belief and to the best of my knowledge, *there is no evidence, empirical or theoretical, that elevating leg rests will reduce LE edema in an individual sitting upright.*[6,21]

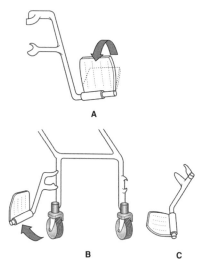

A

B   C

FIGURE 7-26 Front rigging features: **(A)** Flip-up footplates enable access for transfers. **(B)** Swing-away front rigging enables better access for transfers but is less durable and adds weight. **(C)** Detachable front rigging improves maneuverability in small spaces.

---

* Elevating leg rests often accompany recliner frames.

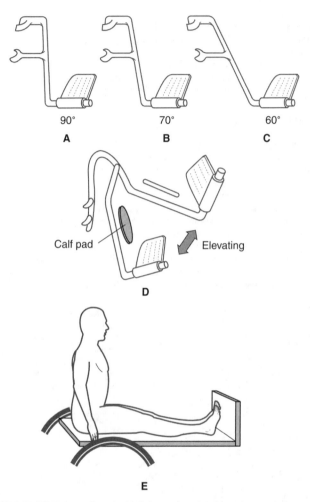

FIGURE 7-27 (A) 90-degree front rigging helps to place tight hamstrings on slack.
(B) Standard front rigging is fixed at 70 degrees. **(C)** 60-degree front rigging provides better caster clearance but increases wheelchair length. **(D)** Elevating leg rests have adjustable angles to enable adjustable limb elevation. **(E)** Custom LE panels elevate and fix the LEs in extension but make transfers difficult.

Angle of Front Rigging

Front rigging can support the LE at various knee angles (Figure 7-27).

- *70 degrees*—A standard support bracket that is fixed and angled at 70 degrees from a horizontal plane.
- *90 degrees*—The support bracket is fixed and angled at 90 degrees from a horizontal plane to provide 90-degree knee flexion while sitting. Hamstrings are placed on slack and knee flexion contractures are accommodated more in 90-degree than in 70-degree brackets.
- *60 degrees*—The support bracket is fixed and angled at 60 degrees from a horizontal plane, thus improving caster clearance but increasing overall wheelchair length.[24]
- *Elevating adjustable angle*—The support bracket is adjustable and elevates or lowers the limb. The length of the support bracket will need to be adjusted following changes in the angle of elevation.
- *Fixed angle*—Nonadjustable custom panels support the LEs when knees are fixed in extension. A nonadjustable, fixed angle panel can interfere with transfers and will increase the overall length and weight of the wheelchair.

Footplates and Supports (Footrests)

Footplates provide a support surface for the feet and can range from simple standard foot plates to a custom footbox configuration (Figure 7-28).

- *Standard footplates*—Each foot is supported in a neutral ankle position.
- *One-piece footboard*—If the patient is strong and tends to break footplates, consider installing a one-piece footboard across both footplates to strengthen foot support, or request reinforcing the footplates with hardware or welding. (Note that welding renders the attachment permanent and nonadjustable.)

  - More stable surface[3]
  - Larger foot support area
  - May increase support strength
  - Can be swing-away for transfers (if not welded)
  - May interfere with independent transfers
  - Adds weight to frame

- *Footplate extenders*—If the footplates are located too far forward relative to the feet or the patient has knee flexion contractures, consider extending the footplates posteriorly and under the wheelchair using footplate extenders so feet are adequately supported.
- *Foot sandals*—If the patient's feet need to remain positioned but are difficult to stabilize with straps, consider foot sandals. Sandals provide greater contact and support by surrounding the border of each foot and securing the foot down with straps.
- *Adjustable angle footplates*—If the ankles are fixed in dorsiflexion or plantarflexion, consider angle-adjustable footplates to accommodate the deformity.

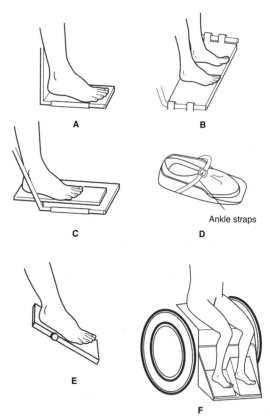

FIGURE 7-28 Footplates and supports: **(A)** Standard footplates. **(B)** A one-piece footboard offers greater stability and surface area. **(C)** Footplate extenders help accommodate hamstring tightness. **(D)** Foot sandals provide a secure foot placement. **(E)** Angled footplates accommodate limited foot and ankle range. **(F)** A custom footbox accommodates bilateral LE asymmetry.

- *Custom footbox*—If the patient has fixed LE deformity resulting in foot locations that cannot be supported by conventional front rigging, consider a custom footbox that can provide individual support for each foot. Footboxes add substantial weight to the wheelchair.

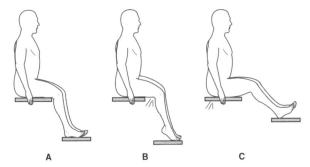

FIGURE 7-29 (A) Adequate footplate height without excessive pressures under thigh or buttocks. **(B)** If footplate is adjusted too low, excessive pressure at distal posterior thigh and forward pelvic sliding can occur. **(C)** If footplate is adjusted too high, excessive ischial pressure, heel pressure, and pressure sores can occur.

Footplate Height

The footplate should support the weight of the lower limb and allow the thighs to rest parallel to the seat surface without excessive pressure distally under the thigh or proximally under the buttocks (Figure 7-29).

- *If footplates are too low*, the feet may hang, causing excessive pressure under the distal thighs, resulting in restricted circulation.[2] The patient may also slide forward in the seat.
- *If footplates are too high*, so the distal thigh no longer contacts the seat, excessive ischial pressure and potential ulcer development at the ischia, coccyx, or sacrum may result.

Leg Rest Support and Test Dummy Stability

Some evidence suggests that use of leg rest support (and seat belts) on power chairs helps prevent instability and falling episodes when obstacles such as ascending curbs (at a 45-degree approach), curb cuts, and descending 5-degree ramps are encountered. Instability in test dummies increased when leg rests were not in use. Generalizability is limited, of course, because chairs were not evaluated with human subjects.[51]

Comments

- *If the patient wears shoes with braces*, make sure the footplates are large enough.
- *If footplates are low to the floor*, they may interfere with the casters' capability to rotate. Family members may complain that the wheelchair does not turn. Consider smaller casters or 60-degree support brackets if the patient has sufficient hamstring length, to address caster clearance problems.

- Avoid having the front rigging put pressure on the patient's peroneal nerve at the level of the fibula head.
- Patients and caregivers tend to trip over front rigging if it cannot be removed during transfers. To avoid accidents, consider swing-away, detachable features (Figure 4-2).
- Elevating leg rests are heavier than footrests, can make the wheelchair longer, and could shift the center of gravity of the wheelchair forward when elevated, thereby making it easier to tip the frame forward. These devices should not be used to stretch tight hamstrings.

Heel Loops

Heel loops are nonrigid semicircular-shaped material located on the rear portion of the footplate behind the patient's heel (Figure 1-1).

Indication

- To prevent the feet from falling behind the footplates

Comments

- Consider stiffer heel loop material if heel loops lose their shape and flatten down over time.
- If the patient's feet fall behind the footplate with heel loops in use, consider a higher (i.e., taller) heel loop, a calf strap, or a calf panel, or construct a back wall for the footplate.
- If the patient vigorously lifts and lowers the foot onto the footplate (stomps feet), make sure hardware (i.e., bolts) that secures the heel loops to the footrest will not cause injury to the foot.

Ankle Straps

Ankle straps are small belts that secure the foot and ankle to the footplates (Figure 7-28D).

Advantages

- Prevent the foot from falling off the footplate
- Maintain flexed lower limb alignment of the ankle and knee in the wheelchair
- Position LEs in patients with significant spasticity[10]

Disadvantages

- Limit freedom of movement (i.e., kicking movements)
- Interfere with independent transfers

Comments

- An ankle strap angle at 45 degrees encourages pressure toward the heel and may help to inhibit a support reaction.[4]
- Strong patients may break through Velcro-secured straps. Consider belt buckles with leather straps for strong patients, but make sure the metal buckle either does not cause skin pressure or is properly padded.
- Ankle straps function best and will probably be tolerated better if the patient wears shoes or sneakers rather than socks or bare feet.
- Ankle straps should be long enough to fit around the patient's shoes containing braces.
- Patients with LE flexor activity may slide forward in the wheelchair if ankle straps are used because they will attempt to pull up their feet, which are anchored to the footplates.

Calf Pad

A calf pad is a flat rigid cushioned support located on the front rigging (i.e., elevating leg rests) at the level of the calf (Figure 7-27D, Figure 6-6).

Advantage

- Physical support for the calf when the leg rest is elevated.[2]

Comment

- Calf pads are primarily used on elevating leg rests.

Calf Strap

A calf strap is a nonrigid support suspended across the support bracket of the front rigging and is situated behind the patient's calf (Figure 1-1).

Advantage

- Discourages the feet from falling behind the footplates and under the wheelchair. Calf straps may be useful in patients with LE flexor activity or patients who do not tolerate heel loops and ankle straps.

Disadvantage

- May interfere with the ability of front rigging to swing away

Rear Antitippers

Rear antitippers (antitipper extensions)[26] are metal tubes with small wheels that attach to the rear of the wheelchair frame near the floor (Figure 7-30, Figure 6-2).

FIGURE 7-30 Rear antitippers protect users from backward tips but can interfere with curb negotiation.

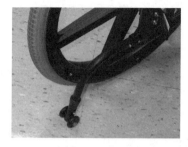

Indication

- Use for safety to prevent the wheelchair from tipping backward.[2] Rear antitippers are a popular solution for instability resulting when wheelchairs are configured with rear wheels placed forward (to promote energy-efficient propulsion).[47]

Disadvantages

- Can interfere with mobility (i.e., popping a wheelie) and curb negotiation in active wheelchair users.
- Tend to get lost easily if detached from wheelchair.
- Tend to easily break if people step on them (in order to raise front wheels up a curb). See Figure 11-2.
- Caregivers who push wheelchair may bang the front of their legs into antitippers. Warn the caregivers ahead of time.

Comments

- An alternative patented self-deployable arc rear antitip device, designed to permit additional rear tipping, has been evaluated by its inventor.[52]
- Caregivers should not step down on antitippers to go up curbs. They easily break. Use the short tipping level for this purpose.
- Wheelchair-related fatalities are associated with wheelchair tipping.[30]
- Antitippers are useful, but they don't work unless they are pointed downward. Keep them pointed down toward the floor except for going up curbs.
- If the patient tends to tip the wheelchair forward, consider front antitippers, which attach to the front of the frame. Front antitippers may interfere during ramp and curb negotiation, however.
- If the patient tends to tip the wheelchair sideways, you have a problem. Sideways antitippers are not common. Consider widening the wheelchair's base of support by cambering the rear wheels, adding another wheel, or thicker

wheel, or getting a wider frame if absolutely necessary. Even then, the patient should be monitored. I've observed a few patients with Huntington's chorea tip wheelchairs over regardless of efforts to prevent it.

Short Tipping Lever

The short tipping lever is tubing on the rear of the frame, near the floor, that the caregiver steps down on with one foot in order to raise the front wheels (i.e., caster) in the air to negotiate curbs. Use these levers and not antitippers to raise casters.[26]

Push Handles

Push handles may be optional, but are required for attendant-operated wheelchairs. Independent, active wheelchair users may find push handles degrading (see Figure 1-1, Figure 6-2).[10]

Storage, Holders, and Poles

- *Utility bags*—If the patient needs to carry medically related supplies (e.g., diapers, chucks, medication), consider ordering a bag to hang from the rear of the wheelchair. Be aware that placing a bag or backpack over the back of the wheelchair can decrease the backward stability of the chair.[53]
- *Underseat pouches*—An underseat pouch can be convenient for storing small items while avoiding some of the center of gravity backward stability issues of utility bags.[53]
- *Crutch and cane holders (carrier)*—For patients who can ambulate short distances with a cane or crutch, consider a holder that stores the device in an upright position.[53]
- *Oxygen tank holders*—For patients who require oxygen while traveling in a wheelchair, make sure to match the correct oxygen tank holder with oxygen cylinder size.
- *Feeding poles*—If the patient is being continuously fed through a tube, consider attaching a feeding pole attachment.
- *IV pole extensions*—For patients taking IV medications, a pole extension attached to the wheelchair to hang the fluid bag would be convenient.
- *Ventilation (vent) racks*—For patients on a vent, anticipate its storage and placement requirements on the wheelchair.

EXERCISE

Go to the Internet and get a "ball park" price range for foam, gel, and air cushions. What does a custom molded insert cost?

References

1. Trefler E, Hobson DA, Taylor SJ, Monahan LC, Shaw CG. *Seating and Mobility for Persons with Physical Disabilities*. Tucson, AZ: Therapy Skill Builders; 1993:242–248.
2. Wilson AB, Mcfarland SR. Types of wheelchairs. *J Rehabil Res Dev*. 1990;2(Supp):104–116.
3. Bergen AF, Presperin J, Tallman T. *Positioning for Function: Wheelchairs and Other Assistive Technologies*. Valhalla, NY: Valhalla Rehabilitation; 1990:13–82.
4. Taylor SJ. Evaluating the client with physical disabilities for wheelchair sitting. *Am J Occup Ther*. 1987;41:711–716.
5. Harrymann SE, Warren LR. Positioning and power mobility. In Church G, Glennen S, eds. *The Handbook of Assistive Technologies*. San Diego: Singular; 1992:55–92.
6. Sabol TP, Haley ES. Wheelchair evaluation for the older adult. *Clin Geriatr Med*. 2006;22:355–375.
7. Jarvis S. Wheelchair clinics for children. *Physiother*. 1985;71:132–134.
8. Brubaker C. Ergonometric considerations. *J Rehabil Res Dev*. 1990;2(Supp):37–48.
9. Grunewald J. Wheelchair selection from a nursing perspective. *Rehabil Nurs*. 1986;11:31–32.
10. Currie DM, Hardwick K, Marburger RA, Britell CW. Wheelchair prescription and adaptive seating. In Delisa JL, Gans BM, eds. *Rehabilitation Medicine: Principles and Practice*. 2nd ed. Philadelphia: J B Lippincott; 1993:563–585.
11. Garber SL. Classification of wheelchair cushions. *Am J Occup Ther*. 1979;10:652–654.
12. Van der Woude LH, Veeger D-J, Rozendal RH. Seat height in handrim wheelchair propulsion. *J Rehabil Res Dev*. 1989;26(4):31–50.
13. Batavia AI, Batavia AI. Pressure ulcer in a man with tetraplegia and a poorly fitting wheelchair: a case report with clinical and policy implications. *Spinal Cord*. 1999;37(2):140–141.
14. Maurer CL, Sprigle S. Effect of seat inclination on seated pressures of individuals with spinal cord injury. *Phys Ther*. 2004;84(3):255–261.
15. Garber SL, Krouskop TA, Carter RE. A system for clinically evaluating wheelchair pressure-relief cushions. *Am J Occup Ther*. 1978;32(9):565–570.
16. Garber SL. Wheelchair cushions: a historical review. *Am J Occup Ther*. 1985;39:453–459.
17. Walls G. Choosing the right cushion. *Rehab Manage*. 2002;15(1):32–36.
18. Brienza DM, Geyer MJ. Using support surfaces to manage tissue integrity. *Adv Skin Wound Care*. 2005;18(3):151–157.
19. Kurfuerst S, Chew F. Cushion conclusions. *Rehab Manage*. 2003;16(7):52–56.
20. Ferguson-Pell MW. Seat cushion selection. *J Rehabil Res Dev*. 1990;2(Supp):49–73.
21. Paleg G. Pediatric seating and support. *Rehab Manage*. 2006;19(1):55–56,58–59.
22. Stockton L, Rithalia S. Is dynamic seating a modality worth considering in the prevention of pressure ulcers? *J Tissue Viability*. 2007;17:15–21.
23. Sprigle S. Categorizing cushions. *Rehab Manage*. 2004;17(3):28–30, 32.
24. Kohlmeyer KM, Yarkony GM. Functional outcomes after spinal cord injury rehabilitation: wheelchairs. In Yarkony GM, ed. *Spinal Cord Injury: Medical Management and Rehabilitation*. Gaithersburg, MD: Aspen; 1994:9–14.

25. Cullum NA, McInnes E, Bell-Syer SEM, Legood R. Support surfaces for pressure ulcer prevention. *Cochrane Database of Systematic Reviews.* 2004, Issue 3. Art. No.: CD001735. DOI: 10.1002/14651858.CD001735.pub2.

26. Ragnarsson KT. Clinical perspectives on wheelchair selection: prescription considerations and a comparison of conventional and lightweight wheelchairs. *J Rehabil Res Dev.* 1990;2(Supp):8–16.

27. Panel for the Prediction and Prevention of Pressure Ulcers in Adults. *Pressure Ulcers in Adults: Prediction and Prevention. Clinical Practice Guideline*, Number 3. Rockville, Md: Agency for Heath Care Policy and Research, Public Health Service, U.S. Department of Health and Human Services; May 1992:26. AHCPR Pub No. 92-0047.

28. Redford JB. Seating and wheeled mobility in the disabled elderly population. *Arch Phys Med Rehabil.* 1993;74:877–885.

29. Holmes KJ, Michael SM, Thorpe SL, Solomonidis SE. Management of scoliosis with special seating for the non-ambulant spastic cerebral palsy population—a biomechanical study. *Clin Biomechan.* 2003;18:480–487.

30. Calder CJ, Kirby RL. Fatal wheelchair-related accidents in the United States. *Am J Phys Med Rehabil.* 1990;69:184-190.

31. Rubin BS, Dube AH, Mitchell EK. Asphyxial deaths due to physical restraint: a case series. *Arch Fam Med.* 1993;2:405–408.

32. Gilsdorf P, Patterson R, Fisher S. Thirty-minute continuous sitting force measurements with different support surfaces in the spinal cord injured and able-bodied. *J Rehabil Res Dev.* 1991;28(4):33–38.

33. McLauin CA, Brubaker CE. Biomechanics and the wheelchair. *Prosthet Orthot Int.* 1991;15:24–37.

34. Brant J. Wheelchair clinics work. *Occup Ther Health Care.* 1988;5:67–70.

35. Warren CG. Technical considerations: power mobility and its implications. *J Rehabil Res Dev.* 1990;2(Supp):74–85.

36. Mattingly D. Wheelchair selection. *Orthop Nurs.* 1993;12:11–17.

37. Ada L, Foongchomcheay A, Canning C. Supportive devices for preventing and treating subluxation of the shoulder after stroke. *Cochrane Database of Systemic Reviews.* (1)CD003863, 2005.

38. Kamenetz HL. *The Wheelchair Book: Mobility for the Disabled.* Springfield, CT: CC Thomas; 1969:132–134.

39. American Academy of Pediatrics. Policy statement. February and May 2008. Available at: http://aappolicy.aappublications.org/cgi/content/full/pediatrics;122/2/450. Accessed November 6, 2008.

40. Everest & Jennings Inc. *Wheelchair Prescription: Care and Service* (Booklet no. 4). Los Angeles, CA: Everest & Jennings, Inc. 1976; 8.

41. Simmons SF, Schnelle JF, MacRae PG, Ouslander JG. Wheelchairs as mobility restraints: predictors of wheelchair activity in nonambulatory nursing home residence. *J Am Geriatr Soc.* 1995;43(4):384–388.

42. Trudel G, Kirby RL, Ackroyd-Stolarz SA, Kirland S. Effects of rear-wheel camber on wheelchair stability. *Arch Phys Med Rehabil.* 1997;78:78–81.

43. Perdios A, Sawatzky BJ, Sheel AW. Effects of camber on wheeling efficiency in the experienced and inexperienced wheelchair user. *J Rehabil Res Dev.* 2007;44(3):459–466.

44. Behrman, AL. Clinical perspectives on wheelchair selection: factors in functional assessment. *J Rehabil Res Dev.* 1990;2(Supp):17–27.

45. Sawatzky B, Denison I. Wheeling efficiency: the effects of varying tyre pressure with children and adolescents. *Pediatr Rehabil.* 2006;9(2):122–126.

46. Sawatzky BJ, Kim WO, Denison I. The ergonomics of different tyres and tyre pressure during wheelchair propulsion. *Ergonom.* 2004;47(14):1475–1483.
47. Boninger ML, Baldwin M, Cooper RA, Koontz A, Chan L. Manual wheelchair push-rim biomechanics and axle position. *Arch Phys Med Rehabil.* 2000;81(5):608–613.
48. Richter WM, Rodriguez R, Woods KR, Karpinski AP, Axelson PW. Reduced finger and wrist flexor activity during propulsion with a new flexible handrim. *Arch Phys Med Rehabil.* 2006;87:1643–1647.
49. Hillman M. Wheelchair wheels for use on sand. *Med Engineer Phys.* 1994;16:243–247.
50. Cooper RA, Robertson RN, Lawrence B, et al. Life-cycle analysis of depot versus rehabilitation manual wheelchairs. *J Rehabil Res Dev.* 1996;33(1):45–55.
51. Corfman TA, Cooper RA, Fitzgerald SG, Cooper R. Tips and falls during electric-powered wheelchair driving: effects of seatbelt use, legrests, and driving speed. *Arch Phys Med Rehabil.* 2003;84:1797–1802.
52. Kirby RL, Corkum CG, Smith C, Rushton P, MacLeod DA, Webber A. Comparing performance of manual wheelchair skills using new and conventional rear anti-tip devices: randomized controlled trial. *Arch Phys Med Rehabil.* 2008;89:480–485.
53. Cohen D. Optional but necessary. *Rehab Manage.* 2005;18(10):26, 28–29.

PART IV

Ethics, Funding, Documentation, and Fitting

CHAPTER 8

Ethical Issues

Several topics relating to fairness have been covered in the wheelchair prescription literature. The clinician should be aware of these ethical issues prior to ordering.

Patients

Informed Consent: Is the Patient "in the Loop"?

The patient, family, and/or caregiver should be involved in the wheelchair prescription process and the rationale for the prescription from the start. Involving the patient in the process can also improve compliance later.[1] Problems occur when key figures in the patient's life are not present during the evaluation. The benefits as well as the risks of the order should be discussed, and alternative options explored. Should the patient or family oppose recommendations, much time and energy is saved by halting the order and paperwork.

In a Canadian qualitative study of the wheelchair procurement process, one community-dwelling adult with cerebral palsy said about the process: "I wasn't given options about what kind of chair I could have. I was treated like a passive wheelchair occupant rather than an active participant in the process."[1(p170)]

Equipment Tradeoffs

Prescribing equipment will result in some patient benefits as well as some unavoidable disadvantages. A few examples: Providing a postural support system will improve body alignment but at the cost of increasing wheelchair weight. Moving the rear wheels anteriorly in a manual wheelchair will improve pushrim performance but will also increase backward instability of the wheelchair. Ordering a tilt-in-space frame can reduce sitting pressures but at a cost of increased social isolation (looking up at the ceiling). Be aware of tradeoffs (they are omnipresent), and decide on any compromises with the patient.

Gatekeeping: When Is It Fair to Order a New Chair?

Clinicians often play the role of gatekeeper when deciding if a new wheelchair should be ordered. Ethics, a branch of philosophy that addresses fairness, can help clinicians deal with this wheelchair decision. Modern ethics recognizes two opposing schools of thought: *the rights of the individual* versus the *greatest good of everyone (society).*[2]

The Rights of the Individual

Clinicians and families need to consider the rights of patients to reach their fullest functional potential, and to minimize the likelihood of illness (morbidity) and death (mortality). The guiding question is:

> *Will a new wheelchair meaningfully improve the patient's function and reduce morbidity or mortality?*

If the answer is yes, then the wheelchair can be justified and the rights of the individual advocated. One example would be a power wheelchair that allows safe and independent community mobility for an individual who otherwise would have to rely on others for help (function). A second example would be a gel seat cushion for an individual who lacks sensation and would be at high risk for a pressure ulcer (morbidity). A third example is a wheelchair for a bedridden individual who could aspirate (i.e., choke) and die (of pneumonia) if continually fed in a recumbent position (mortality).

The Greatest Good

On the other hand, considering the needs of the "greatest good" or of society means distributing *limited resources* (funding for wheelchairs) fairly and to those *most in need.* Limited resources, therefore, should not be allocated in excess to any one individual to the extent that these resources are then not available for others in need. A guiding question is:

> *Can the existing wheelchair be used to improve the patient's function and reduce morbidity or mortality?*

If the answer is yes, then it behooves the clinician and family to advocate for the greatest good of society while still addressing the patient's needs. Unnecessarily ordering a wheelchair could result in less funding for others in need, contribute to the national debt of future generations, burden taxpayers, and saturate landfills. An example is a patient who comes to the clinic wanting a new wheelchair because the existing one is 4 years old, but without any other claim. If the wheelchair fits and addresses the medical and functional needs of the patient, then it would be reasonable for third-party payers to question the funding request.

Suppliers

Questionable Practices

In the recent past, suppliers—and some prescribers—committed large-scale Medicare fraud by offering scooters to "patients" who didn't need them and in some cases never received them.[3,4] Red flags[5] of questionable practices include:

(1) suppliers telling patients they know how to get the insurance company to pay for equipment; and (2) suppliers who do not provide services but request the patient's insurance number for their records. Work with reputable suppliers who have memberships in professional organizations and subscribe to a code of ethics.

The following link will be helpful for learning more about Medicare fraud and reporting it: http://www.medicare.gov/FraudAbuse/Tips.asp.

Suppliers: Limited Choices

Make sure your supplier offers a wide range of products and has experience working with your kinds of clients. There is some concern in the literature that competitive bidding (suppliers securing contracts to service durable medical equipment in a given region of the United States) may lead to a limited selection of products for complex clients[6,7] (e.g., lower quality equipment having a greater profit margin) and a less technically trained staff of suppliers to service them.[8]

Manufacturers

Truth in Advertising

The buzz word for manual wheelchairs is weight—that is, very light weight. The lighter the better because heavy chairs roll with greater resistance and require more energy to push. The wheelchair weights listed by manufacturers, however, may not always accurately reflect the total weight delivered to the patient's doorstep;[9] for example, some components may not be included in the calculation. Make sure you are informed of the *actual* wheelchair weight—including all needed components such as leg rests—before ordering.

Disclosure of ANSI/RESNA Wheelchair Standards Test Results

Wheelchair standards provide an objective means for comparison shopping so patients can make informed purchases based on features that are important to them.[10] For one person durability may be most important; for another, stability. Although manufacturer disclosure of American National Standards Institute/Rehabilitation Engineering and Assistive Technology Society of North America (ANSI/RESNA) wheelchair standards test results are voluntary, many have not fully complied in the past, for a number of business-related reasons.[10-12] Full compliance would help consumers (patients) make informed purchasing decisions that are best for their health, lifestyle, and pocketbook.

Public Funding: Medicare's "In the House" Rule

Medicare only considers the medical necessity of equipment for use in the home, despite internal dissent from some of its policy panel members.[13,14] The problem is that the "in the house" rule runs counter to current practical, medical, and world views on health. First, clinicians must consider the reality of *outdoor* challenges when prescribing wheelchairs. A patient who tries to keep medical appointments will encounter multiple hurdles: curbs, steps, poorly maintained sidewalks, street crossings, slopes, and inclement weather, none of which would be a problem within the home. Second, the ruling is inconsistent with current medical literature that documents the deleterious effects of home confinement (i.e., malnutrition, depression, decreased quality of life, increased use of aides).[15] Third, the ruling is out of sync with the World Health Organization's 21st-century International Classification of Functioning, Disability, and Health (ICF) classification that recognizes the importance of societal participation,[14] and thus by extension, visiting the world outside the home.

References

1. Mortenson WB, Miller WC. The wheelchair procurement process: perspective of clients and prescribers. *Can J Occup Ther*. 2008;75(3):167–175.
2. Callihan JC, ed. *Ethical Issues in Professional Life*. New York: Oxford University Press; 1988.
3. Associated Press. Wheelchair scams cost Medicare millions. Available at: http://www.cnn.com/2003/HEALTH/11/11/us.wheelchair.ap. Accessed October 23, 2008.
4. Goodwin JS, Nguyen-Oghalai TU, Kuo Y-F, Ottenbacher KJ. Epidemiology of Medicare abuse: the example of power wheelchairs. *J Am Geriatr Soc*. 2007;55:221–226.
5. Centers for Medicare and Medicaid Services. Medicare fraud: detection and prevention tips. Available at: http://www.medicare.gov/FraudAbuse/Tips.asp. Accessed October 26, 2008.
6. Carlson AH. Power play: Medicare reimbursement cuts for scooters may steer patients to cash-based options. *Rehab Manage*. 2007;20(7):22, 24–25.
7. Margolis S. Access denied: consequences of federal policy on seating and wheeled mobility. *J Rehabil Res Dev*. 2004;41(4): vii–ix.
8. Smith R. Surviving 2006 guidelines. Available at: http://www.rehabpub.com/features/42006/8.asp. Accessed November 13, 2006.
9. Smith ME. Playing the weight game: understanding the whole story behind manual wheelchair weight specifications. Available at: http://www.wheelchairjunkie.com/manualweights.html. Accessed November 5, 2008.
10. Cooper RA. Wheelchair standards: it's all about quality assurance and evidence-based practice. *J Spinal Cord Med*. 2006;29(2):93–94.
11. Cooper RA, Robertson RN, Lawrence B, et al. Life-cycle analysis of depot versus rehabilitation manual wheelchairs. *J Rehabil Res Dev*. 1996;33(1):45–55.
12. Cooper RA, Gonzalez J, Lawrence B, Renschler A, Boninger ML, VanSickle DP. Performance of selected lightweight wheelchairs on ANSI/RESNA tests. American National Standards Institute–Rehabilitation Engineering and Assistive Technology Society of North America. *Arch Phys Med Rehabil*. 1997;78(10):1138–1144.
13. Canning B. Funding, ethics, and assistive technology: should medical necessity be the criterion by which wheeled mobility equipment is justified? *Top Stroke Rehabil*. 2005;12(3):77.
14. Dicianno BE, Tovey E. Power mobility device provision: understanding Medicare guidelines and advocating for clients. *Arch Phys Med Rehabil*. 2007;88:807–816.
15. Medicare Rights Center. Forcing isolation: Medicare's "in the home" coverage standard for wheelchairs. *Care Manag J*. 2005;6(1):29–37.

Funding

Once the patient has been examined, simulated (e.g., trial period), and the equipment decided upon, it's time to get it paid for. Know the patient's funding options.[1] Funding can be divided into four areas:[2,3] public, private, nonprofit/ donations/charity, and self-pay. Each funding source has its own eligibility criteria (who's covered) and rules for coverage (what's covered). Do your homework— don't approach an agency you know will deny coverage. Medicare, for example, will not approve a stair-climbing wheelchair, whereas the Veterans Administration just might.[4] Insurance specialists who work for the wheelchair supply company (if you decide to go with that company) can offer guidance on funding options for their products.[3]

Public Funding

Medicare

Medicare is a federal insurance program that funds persons 65 years of age or older, people with certain disabilities under age 65, and people in end-stage renal disease.[2,3,5,6] Part B of Medicare funds equipment, including wheelchairs, based on medical necessity. To help you understand the rationale for Medicare wheelchair approvals, see Medicare's algorithm in Appendix A. Some points about the algorithm are highlighted below.[7,8]

The Medicare Algorithm

The algorithm is a flow chart that provides guidance for clinical decision making about wheelchair requests.[9] The process is sequential and hierarchical: First determine if an ambulatory aid (such as a cane) will address the patient's in-home mobility-related activities of daily living (ADL) problem; if not, consider manual wheelchairs, then scooters, and finally power wheelchairs.

- "In-the-home" coverage: Medicare is interested in patient mobility-related activities of daily living (MRADLs) limitations for feeding, bathing, dressing, toileting, and grooming in "customary locations" within the home. For example, can the patient perform these activities in the morning in a safe manner and within a reasonable time frame?[10] A limitation can be cited if the patient:

(1) cannot do it at all (inability), (2) cannot do it safely (unsafe), or (3) cannot do it in a timely manner (too time consuming). Mobility aids are then considered to address the limitation in a step-by-step process.

- Funding agencies like Medicare look at 5 years for expected device durability.[11]
- Equipment may be rented or purchased. If rented, the original supplier is responsible for all repairs—you can't go anywhere else for repairs (even if the patient is on vacation elsewhere).
- Only one piece of equipment is generally funded.[1]

Equipment Denials: Some Reasons[7,8]

- Patient not eligible for Medicare part B
- Supplier not enrolled in Medicare
- Wheelchair not coded in Medicare
- Patient displays poor compliance, safety, cognition, or vision for that equipment
- Home not physically accessible
- Assistances required but not available
- Item not judged medically necessary
- Incomplete paperwork submitted (i.e., relevant medical records; timeliness within 45 days of the evaluation)
- Required evaluation not performed (i.e., face-to-face meeting with the practitioner)
- Equipment request is for outside the home (i.e., community use)

Medicaid

Medicaid is a state–federal program offered and managed at the state level; guidelines, services, and eligibility *vary by state*.[3,5,6,12] Eligibility is generally based on being categorically needy, medically needy, or in a special group;[5,12] persons with disabilities probably fall into the second group. A caseworker can evaluate the patient's eligibility for a given state. Like Medicare, Medicaid funding for equipment is often based on medical necessity.

U.S. Department of Veterans Affairs

At the federal level, if a patient is eligible for veteran's benefits, a wheelchair may be provided when it is medically necessary.[2,3,6,13] Benefits can be found through the department's Prosthetics Web page: "What to Expect from Your VA Prosthetic and Sensory Aids Service" (http://www.prosthetics.va.gov/docs/IB-10-62-v3.pdf).

For specific information on manual wheelchair and motorized wheeled mobility device coverage at the VA, click on the Clinical Practice Recommendations at the VA's Prosthetics and Sensory Aids Service page: http://www.prosthetics.va.gov/cpr.asp.

Vocational Rehabilitation

At the state level, if assistive technology such as a wheelchair is needed in connection with work/job training, funding may be available.[2,6]

- To find vocational rehabilitation benefits in a specific state, search online for Vocational Rehabilitation and your state (e.g., Vocational Rehabilitation AND New York).
- Also see http://www.parac.org/srac.html.

Workers' Compensation

If a wheelchair is needed in connection with work-related injuries, workers' compensation benefits may apply.[2] To search for workers' compensation information by state, go to http://www.comp.state.nc.us/ncic/pages/wcadmdir.htm.

Individuals with Disabilities Education Act (IDEA)

If a child, age 3 to 21, with a disability can show that assistive technology such as a wheelchair will increase their ability to obtain appropriate free public education within a least restrictive environment, the school district will provide the equipment in accordance with the Individuals with Disabilities Education Act (IDEA). Equipment is decided on a case-by-case basis.[2,14,15]

- For general information about the Individuals with Disabilities Education Act, go to http://idea.ed.gov.
- For inquiries about submitting assistive technology requests such as wheelchairs, in connection to a student's Individualized Education Plan (IEP), contact the local school district's committee on special education.

Private Funding

Private Insurance

For those patients who have private insurance, either through their job or individually, one needs to carefully *read their policy* to determine which equipment is and is not covered. If covered, approval is often based on the insurance company's definition of medical necessity.[2,6] Private insurance companies may be more willing to fund a wheelchair than a public source like Medicare.[1] Nevertheless, gaining approval is not always a piece of cake, even if you're familiar with the health care industry.

In the article, "Of Mice and Wheelchairs," Harvard-trained lawyer and health policy professor Andrew I. Batavia describes his trials and tribulations in securing approval for a costly but needed tilt-in-space power chair from his preferred provider organization (PPO). In the excerpt below, Batavia describes how he was caught between the insurance and medical systems' gridlock when attempting to replace his 5- to 6-year-old, deteriorating power chair.

By this time I was beginning to develop conspiracy theories: My physician is unwilling to write a prescription if my PPO is willing to pay to repair the chair, and my PPO is unwilling to pay for a new chair unless my physician is willing to write a prescription for it. A classic Catch-22.[17(pp180–181)]

Nonprofit/Donations/Charity

Nonprofit organizations offer used or refurbished wheelchairs to those in need.[2,3] Because these chairs are old, have been donated, or are repaired, they may not be covered under the manufacturer's warranty. Depending on the organization's policy, the patient may be required to sign a liability release before obtaining the wheelchair. Having the chair inspected by the original manufacturer or a supplier for road-worthiness/safety may be a good idea. For a list of local, national, and international organizations involved in donations, see the links below. Wikipedia and Mobility Adviser both list a number of organizations involved with donation.

Links to Lists of Wheelchair Organizations Involved in Donation

- Wikipedia: http://en.wikipedia.org/wiki/List_of_wheelchair_organizations
- Mobility Advisor: http://www.mobility-advisor.com/wheelchair-donations .html
- Pass It On Center, a national assistive technology reuse center: http://www .passitoncenter.org/index.shtml

Self-Pay

Cash

Suppliers will always take cash. Make sure you get a receipt, all warranty documentation, and contact information. Confirm with third-party payers ahead of time if you plan to be reimbursed for part or all of the purchase cost.

Loans

Loans can of course be secured through banks, but Assistive Technology Loan Programs, which are funded under the Assistive Technology Act of 1998, may offer various competitive loan programs to help persons with disabilities acquire assistive technology that will enhance home/work/school participation.[2]

- Search: Assistive Technology Loan Programs AND your state (e.g., Assistive Technology Loan Programs AND California)
- For technical assistance on state loan programs go to the Alternative Financing Technical Assistance Project at RESNA: http://www.resna.org/projects/ index.php.

References

1. Canning B. Funding, ethics, and assistive technology: should medical necessity be the criterion by which wheeled mobility equipment is justified? *Top Stroke Rehabil.* 2005;12(3):77.
2. ABLEDATA. ABLEDATA informed consumer's guide to funding assistive technology. Available at: http://www.abledata.com/abledata_docs/funding.htm. Accessed November 8, 2008.
3. Buning ME, Schmeler MR, Crane B. Funding for wheelchairs in general. Available at: http://www.wheelchairnet.org/WCN_ProdServ/Funding/funding.html. Accessed September 25, 2006.
4. Department of Veterans Affairs. Clinical practice recommendations for motorized wheeled mobility devices: iBOT power wheelchair. Available at: http://www.prosthetics.va.gov/docs/Motorized_Wheeled_Mobility_Devices_IBOT_Addendum.pdf. Accessed November 6, 2008.
5. Centers for Medicare and Medical Services. Medicaid program general information overview. Available at: http://www.cms.hhs.gov/MedicareGenInfo/. Accessed October 22, 2008.
6. Blake DJ, Bodine C. An overview of assistive technology for persons with multiple sclerosis. *J Rehabil Res Dev.* 2002;39(2):299–312.
7. An algorithmic approach to determine if mobility assistive equipment is reasonable and necessary for Medicare beneficiaries with a personal mobility deficit (CR3791-Mobility Assistive Equipment (MAE)). *MLN Matters;* MM3791; June 3, 2005. Available at: http://www.cms.hhs.gov/MLNMattersArticles/downloads/MM3791.pdf. Accessed January 15, 2008.
8. Brennan S. Medicare coverage for scooters and power wheelchairs national coverage determination for power mobility devices (PMDs). Available at: http://www.phc-online.com/v/vspfiles/html/medicare_coverage_power_mobility.shtml. Accessed October 15, 2008.
9. Dicianno BE, Tovey E. Power mobility device provision: understanding Medicare guidelines and advocating for clients. *Arch Phys Med Rehabil.* 2007;88:807–816.
10. Paleg G. Subject to approval. Available at: http://www.rehabpub.com/issues/articles/2007-01_04.asp. Accessed October 29, 2008.
11. Medicare Rights Center. Forcing isolation: Medicare's "in the home" coverage standard for wheelchairs. *Care Manage J.* 2005;6(1):29–37.
12. Department of Health and Human Services, Centers for Medicare and Medicaid Services. Medicaid at-a-glance 2005: a Medicaid information source. Available at: http://www.cms.hhs.gov/MedicaidDataSourcesGenInfo/02_MAAG2005.asp. Accessed November 11, 2008.
13. Department of Veterans Affairs. Clinical practice recommendations for motorized wheeled mobility devices. Available at: www.prosthetics.va.gov/docs/Motorized_Wheeled_Mobility_Devices.doc. Accessed November 11, 2008.
14. Lance D. The "IDEA" of assistive technology. August 17, 1999. Available at: http://www.suite101.com/print_articlecfm/assistive_technology/24315. Accessed October 23, 2008.
15. Szabo J. School-based physical therapy: what you need to know to get started, part II. *Advance Phys Ther Phys Ther Assist.* 2001;29–30.
16. Golinker L, Mistrett SG. Funding. In Angelo J, ed. *Assistive Technology for Rehabilitation Therapists.* Philadelphia: FA Davis; 1997:211–233.
17. Batavia AI. Of wheelchairs and managed care. *Health Aff.* 1999;18(6):177–182.

CHAPTER 10

Documentation

Reimbursement Letters

Once you identify a funding agency, a reimbursement letter that justifies the equipment request is typically required. The type of justification required will depend on the funding agency. The emphasis may be on educational, job-related, or medically related goals. For Medicare, Medicaid, and most private insurance companies, the justification should be medically related and is referred to as a "letter of medical necessity."

Letter of Medical Necessity

A letter of medical necessity is a document used to medically justify the need for a wheelchair or parts when requesting funding from government and private sources. The letter tells a *story*, incorporating relevant information from the patient's evaluation. In essence, you want to "paint a picture" of how the patient functions (along with limitations) in a typical day.[1] The story should describe the patient's condition, wheelchair-related problems, how these problems impact the patient's condition, and how a new prescription will remedy the patient's mobility problem.

What Is a Medical Necessity?

Unfortunately, no general consensus exists for the term *medical necessity*.[2] It is often associated with "appropriate," "reasonable and necessary," or required to prevent undesirable medical consequences if the equipment is not provided (e.g., deformity, skin ulcer). In most cases, the patient's diagnosis may have some associated risk factors that equipment may help to ameliorate. For example, a person with C4 tetraplegia who, because of paralysis, cannot perform sitting push-ups to relieve pressure may be medically justified in requesting a power tilt mechanism along with a pressure-relieving cushion to fend off an impending pressure ulcer. Thus, relating the request to risk may be fruitful. [2,3]

On the other hand, justification based on expected positive consequences/ benefits, improved quality of life, or recreational need may simply be labeled as "a convenience" by some insurance carriers.[4] Still, the medical necessity of a piece of equipment may be subject to a reviewer's own interpretation of the term, in which case you may have some "wiggle room" to argue your case.[2] For example, you may be able to argue for an ultralight wheelchair with an adjustable rear axle for patients with documented shoulder pain if their ability to self-propel, even indoors, is markedly limited using a heavier, poorly configured standard or light-weight frame.[5] Alternatively, some form of power mobility may better serve the patient with existing upper extremity (UE) pathology.

Know Your Audience

As any good writing teacher will tell you: know your audience. Clinicians should be familiar with the agency's approval criterion and speak to it. For example, Medicare has strict guidelines currently in place.[6,7] (See Appendix A.) The most notorious one is the "in the home" rule.[8] So if you were submitting a funding request to Medicare, the reviewers would be looking for equipment needs related to use in the home—not the community. On the other hand, if you were submitting the identical request to the Veterans Administration, reviewers may wish to know more about the activities the patient engages in within the community (e.g., recreation, sports).[5]

Content of the Letter

Basic items to include in a reimbursement letter are listed below, although the particulars will vary, depending on your target audience.[9,10]

- Date of the evaluation
- Medical diagnosis, body weight, activity level, and relevant past history
- Changes in medical status that may be relevant to the new request (e.g., shoulder pathology and pain with manual wheelchair use)
- Age of any existing wheelchair
- Home accessibility for the equipment in question
- Level of caregiver support
- Any cognitive, judgment, visual impairment, safety, or compliance/motivational issues pertinent to the request
- Clinical impairments, including any issues (e.g., UE pathology, spasticity) that interfere with function
- Functional abilities, including the time frame to complete tasks

  - If the request is to Medicare, include home-related issues in the letter.
  - If the request targets educational funds, include educationally related needs in the letter.
  - If the request targets vocational funds, include job-related requirements in the letter.

- A point by point justification as to why each requested item on the order is needed

- An explanation as to why an alternative, less costly wheelchair or component would not address the patient's needs
- How long the equipment will be needed (for short-term use, rental may be reasonable)

Order of the Letter

The first four paragraphs of the letter generally include background on the patient diagnoses (also past medical history), functional status, clinical status, and social history (including any relevant job or educational history), as they pertain to the patient's wheelchair needs. When possible, quantify descriptions of patients and their situation[1] (e.g., "grade 3 pressure ulcer measuring 4 mm in diameter"; not "a bed sore"; "ambulates 10 feet in 3.5 minutes"; not "ambulates slowly").

In the fifth paragraph, the letter should describe problems with the existing wheelchair (if there is one). In the sixth paragraph, describe the trial/simulation of the patient in the new wheelchair along with outcomes. Finally, recommend the new wheelchair or parts, with justification of every component. Importantly, justify why less costly alternative components or equipment would not be appropriate for this patient. It may be a good idea to support your justification with evidence-based literature.[11,12] Surprisingly, in Guerette et al.'s national survey of pediatric power wheelchair providers, funding requests included evidence-based literature only 17% of the time.[13]

In the closing paragraph, reemphasize why the wheelchair recommended is medically (or educationally, or vocationally) necessary for this patient.

Supplementary Information

Additional documentation can include letters of support from related medical and educational institutions (e.g., occupational therapist [OT], physical therapist [PT], speech therapist, orthopedist, neurologist, pediatrician, school), and relevant information from the patient's medical chart. (Medicare now requires some portions of the medical chart be included in the funding request.) Photographs and videotape (obtain patient consent) illustrating the patient's problem or potential may also help to sway funders. Remarkably, according to the national survey of pediatric power wheelchair providers, funding requests only included videotapes of power wheelchair–driving performance 7% of the time.[13]

If a fire destroyed equipment, send documentation from the fire department. If a theft occurred, send documentation from the police department. If equipment was lost or destroyed by an airline, obtain documentation from the carrier. Follow up with a second letter to the funding source if additional information is requested. If the request for funding is denied and you believe the decision unjust, request an appeal. Finally, if all else fails, find out how to request a fair hearing.

As a practical matter, inquire as to what format the funding agency prefers. You don't want to waste precious time waiting for approval, only to find out you didn't dot an "i" or cross a "t." Although a few funding agencies may accept a brief prescription (Figure 10-1), a checklist (Figure 10-2), or even a table format (Figure 10-3), many expect a cogent letter written in prose style (Figure 10-4). The sample letter in Figure 10-4 is by no means the only route to writing a reimbursement letter. Its purpose is merely to demonstrate the logical flow of information from patient presentation to paper.

To Whom It May Concern,

Jane Doe is a 16-year-old female with spastic quadriplegia cerebral palsy. Please approve an adult tilt-in-space frame with postural supports and a gel cushion.

Sincerely yours,

John Doe, MD

FIGURE 10-1 The brief prescription .

To Whom It May Concern,

Jane Doe is a 16-year-old female with spastic quadriplegia cerebral palsy. Please approve an adult tilt-in-space frame with postural supports and a gel cushion for the following reasons:

☑ Frame outgrown

☑ Frame more than 5 years old

☐ Medical condition changed

☑ Components worn _____ cushion _____

Sincerely yours,

John Doe, MD

FIGURE 10-2 The checklist.

To Whom It May Concern,

Jane Doe is a 16-year-old female with spastic quadriplegia cerebral palsy. Please approve the following items listed in the table.

Sincerely,

John Doe, MD

Equipment	Justification
Gel x seat cushion	Increased risk for ulcers; stable sitting base
Tilt-in-space frame	Unable to weight shift; poor positioning while upright; forward sliding in wheelchair

FIGURE 10-3 The table format.

The Clinic
XYZ Avenue
New York, NY 33333
Phone 212 123-4567

To: ABC Funding Agency
Re: Jane Smith: Letter of Medical Necessity for a New Wheelchair
Chart # 98765
DOB: xx/xx/xx
Funding No # SN0000N

01/15/10

To Whom It May Concern,

(A) Jane Smith is a 16-year-old female with a diagnosis of cerebral palsy (spastic quadriplegia) and profound mental retardation.

Functional Status

Functionally, Jane Smith is nonambulatory, dependent in all activities of daily living, and requires total support to sit and transfer (two-person lifts). She has no functional use of her upper extremities, does not perform independent pressure relief, does not self-propel her wheelchair, and cannot operate power mobility. Jane Smith therefore relies on caregivers to transport her.

(B) **Clinical Status**

Jane is 5 feet 4 inches in height and weighs 110 lbs. She is motorically inactive, and presents with high LE extensor tone, poor sitting balance, and no righting or equilibrium reactions. Posturally, she presents with a forward head, a flexible kyphotic trunk, and sacral sitting due to forward sliding of her pelvis in her chair She cannot lift her trunk and head against gravity and as a result, she tends to look down to the floor when sitting. Upper extremity range is within normal limits. Lower extremity range of motion is within functional limits for sitting with 90° hip flexion, full hip abduction, neutral rotation, 60° popliteal angles, and neutral angles (0°) bilaterally. Her hip-to-hip seat width measures 16.5 inches and she has a 1.5-inch leg length discrepancy (left side shortening). Skin is intact although pressure (redness) is noted over her greater trochanters and under both ischia, which have little soft tissue protection. Jane lacks bowel and bladder control and wears diapers.

Social History

Jane lives with her two parents and three siblings in a ranch-style home that is fully wheelchair accessible. All doorways and hallways have 30- and 36-inch clearances, respectively, and there is a permanent ramp installed at the front entrance. She spends at least 8 hours of her day in her wheelchair that she utilizes for both positioning and transportation to clinic, school, and the park. Her family owns a wheelchair-accessible van but she also travels on the school bus. Her parents are her primary caregivers and are available and physically capable of assisting in all her transfer and transport needs.

(C) **Existing Wheelchair**

Jane Smith's existing standard wheelchair (16" wide x 16" deep) is 5 years old and no longer provides adequate (1) width, (2) postural support, and (3) pressure relief.

(1) The wheelchair is too narrow for Jane. Her mother reports significant weight gain (20 lbs) and growth since Jane received her wheelchair 5 years ago (see attached

FIGURE 10-4 Sample letter of medical necessity for a new wheelchair. Shaded areas highlight important elements in the letter. **(A)** The patient's diagnosis; **(B)** the patient's functional/clinical status and social situation (accessibility and support); **(C)** current wheelchair status, including the age of the wheelchair, if there is one, and detail on all equipment-related problems.

nurse note). She is developing red pressure areas over her greater trochanters because the 16-inch-wide chair is too narrow for her 16.5-inch-wide hip-to-hip body dimension. Remaining in the existing narrow wheelchair may lead to *ulcer development* due to excessive pressure of her greater trochanters against the inside panels of the armrests. A wider wheelchair frame (18 inches) that will accommodate her seat width, clothing, and any future growth is therefore medically necessary.

(2) The existing wheelchair no longer provides sufficient postural support. Jane Smith has poor sitting and can no longer tolerate upright sitting in her standard wheelchair frame. Her school teacher reports that Jane has difficulty participating in class activities because her face is constantly pointed down toward the floor (see attached letter from teacher). Poor sitting balance and poor head control contribute to her forward head, collapsing (kyphotic) trunk, and forward listing trunk. Her extensor hypertonicity contributes to the forward sliding of her pelvis while in the wheelchair. The use of a chest harness has been poorly tolerated and its use has become a major safety hazard. On April 4 of this year, she was found in the hallway, poorly positioned with her neck caught on the top of her chest harness (see attached incident report). Unfortunately, her existing standard frame cannot tilt backwards to provide the gravity-assisted postural support that she needs. Jane Smith therefore requires a backward tilt-in-space frame that will offer safe, gravity-assisted postural support and minimize patient reliance on anterior trunk supports.

(3) The existing foam cushion is 2 years old, is completely worn (i.e., "bottomed out"), and no longer provides comfort or pressure reduction. As a result, she is beginning to show signs of skin tissue compromise at the ischia and cries if she sits longer than 30 minutes.

Evaluation of New Wheelchair

Jane Smith was evaluated at the ABC Seating Clinic in a wider (18" wide x 16" deep), backward tilt-in-space wheelchair frame with a gel cushion on 01/10/10. During simulation, she tolerated the backward tilt (25 degrees) with good head and trunk alignment, no anterior listing of the trunk, and no forward pelvic sliding for a 90-minute duration (see enclosed photographs). Her mother reported that she was more comfortable (i.e., she fell asleep during part of the evaluation) and her school teacher reports it was easier for Jane to socialize and participate in class activities while in the tilted position. At the conclusion of the evaluation, skin was inspected and no erythema (i.e., redness) were noted at her hips or ischia.

Wheelchair Recommendations

A new wheelchair with a manual backward tilt-in-space frame is recommended to accommodate Jane Smith's body dimensions, postural alignments, and pressure relief needs. These problems can no longer be addressed with her existing standard wheelchair. Although we considered a less costly alternative—a semi-reclining wheelchair frame— forward sliding with accompanying shear forces would unfortunately continue to be a problem. As reported by Hobson, reclining reduced sitting pressures in a group of wheelchair users with paralysis, but it also led to a 25% rise in shear forces.

FIGURE 10-4 (continued) **(D)** supportive documentation (e.g., reference to school nurse and teacher attachments); **(E)** simulation and outcome; **(F)** overall wheelchair recommendations and consideration of alternative less costly solutions; **(G)** cited medical evidence (literature) supporting the need for a component (e.g., tilt-in space feature; pneumatic casters);

(continues)

Mobility Base—(Brand X) Backward Tilt-in-Space Wheelchair—to provide aggressive gravity-assisted postural support and to redistribute pressure. Henderson et al. found that a 65-degree backward tilt significantly reduced ischial pressure an average of 47% in persons with SCI.

- **Size**: Adult size (18" W x 16" D) to accommodate anthropometrics, clothing, and future growth of this 16-year-old patient
- **Front rigging**: Standard 70-degree front rigging secondary to full ROM
- **Armrests**: Adjustable height, removable, full-length armrests—to support a lap board, provide an appropriate UE support level for school activities, and facilitate two-person transfer activities
- **Wheel locks**: Attendant-operated toggle locks for operation by the caregiver. Wheel locks are necessary for safety during transfer activities.
- **Rear wheels**: 24-inch diameter spokeless (mag) wheels with pneumatic tires for shock absorption/comfortable ride for use outdoors, to school, and to the park. Jane's parents are capable of maintaining proper tire air pressure and repairing any flats.
- **Casters**: Large 8-inch diameter casters with pneumatic tires to facilitate negotiation over cracks and objects outdoors. Pneumatic casters may help extend the life of the frame. A study by Cooper et al. found that rehabilitation wheelchairs with pneumatic casters that were fatigue tested using ANSI/RESNA wheelchair standards lasted 3 times longer than the same chair models tested using 8-inch solid casters.

Postural Support System

- **Seat insert**: Split seat insert with mild curve (shorter on left side) to accommodate a 1.5-inch shorter left femur and provide more contact points to distribute pressure under the buttocks
- **Seat cushion**: Gel cushion (F brand). Gel material is easy to clean, offers a stable sitting surface, and was tolerated well during the evaluation. (Pressure areas were previously noted with foam cushion.) Pressure reduction in this client is necessary due to high risk of pressure sore development (inactivity, incontinence, underweight).
- **Cushion covers**: Two incontinence covers—to facilitate cleaning and protect cushion from feces and urine due to client incontinence
- **Back insert**: Planar-shaped back insert with shoulder height to provide necessary spinal support due to poor sitting balance
- **Trunk supports**:
  - **Curved lateral trunk supports**: To discourage lateral trunk listing due to poor trunk control and promote vertical alignment of the trunk in the coronal plane. Curved supports will provide greater points of contact for this low tone client.
  - **Chest belt**: To discourage anterior trunk listing. Adequate clearance will be measured for her neck.
- **Head support**: Curved headrest with an occipital ridge—to address poor head control and encourage midline position of client's head. An occipital ridge can help discourage hyperextension of the client's head.
- **Seat belt**: Auto seat belt with a 2-inch width, positioned at a 45-degree angle to maintain proper pelvic positioning, to prevent forward sliding of the pelvis, and for safety during transportation

FIGURE 10-4 (continued) **(H)** mobility base with medical justification; **(I)** postural support system with medical justification; **(J)** seat cushion justification based on risk factors associated with the diagnosis;

- **Transit option**: So wheelchair will be WC 19 compliant during school bus transportation
- **Ankle straps**: Velcro straps to maintain feet on footplates
- **Heel loops**: To maintain proper placement of feet on footplates and prevent feet from falling posteriorly off footrests
- **Lap board**: For UE support, for programming activities at school, and for support during eating at school and home
- **Protraction blocks**: Attached to the lap board to prevent the client's UEs from falling behind the board while the wheelchair is in a backward tilt position
- **Antitippers**: For safety from backward instability when the chair is tilted backward

Accessories:

- **Air pump**: To maintain sufficient air pressure in pneumatic tires

In summary, we recommend an 18-inch-wide backward tilt-in-space wheelchair system (model # ZZZ) with a gel cushion as a medical necessity to discourage postural deformity and prevent the incidence of pressure ulcer development in this patient with spastic quadriplegia. We anticipate this equipment will be needed on a long-term basis.

Thank you for your attention regarding Jane Smith and our recommendation for a new wheelchair. Please contact us for any additional information.

Sincerely yours,
Mitchell Batavia PhD, PT
John Doe MD

References

Cooper RA, Robertson RN, Lawrence B, et al. Life-cycle analysis of depot versus rehabilitation manual wheelchairs. *J Rehabil Res Dev.* 1996;33(1):45–55.

Henderson JL, Price SH, Brandstater ME, Mandac BR. Efficacy of three measures to relieve pressure in seated persons with spinal cord injury. *Arch Phys Med Rehabil.* 1994;75:535–539.

Hobson DA. Comparative effects of posture on pressure and shear at the body-seat interface. *J Rehabil Res Dev.* 1992;29(4):21–31.

FIGURE 10-4 (continued) **(K)** summary, reiterating medically related need for the equipment (e.g., discourage deformity and pressure ulcers); **(L)** reference list of cited medical literature.

EXERCISE

1. Letter of medical necessity

    a. What major headings would you include in a letter of medical necessity?

    b. How could you further substantiate the medical necessity of a wheelchair for a client who was denied funding?

References

1. Brennan S. Medicare coverage for scooters and power wheelchairs coverage determination for power mobility devices (PMDs). Available at: http://www.phconline.com/v/vspfiles/html/medicare_coverage_power_mobility.shtml. Accessed October 15, 2008.

2. Canning B. Funding ethics, and assistive technology: should medical necessity be the criterion by which wheeled mobility equipment is justified? *Top Stroke Rehabil.* 2005;12(3):77.

3. Cohen D. Optional but necessary. *Rehab Manag.* 2005;18(10):26,28–29.

4. Centers for Medicare and Medicaid Services. Protecting Medicare's power wheelchair and scooter benefit. Available at: http://www.medicare.gov/Publications/Pubs/pdf/11046.pdf. Accessed November 13, 2008.

5. Paleg G. Not a lightweight decision. *Rehab Manag.* 2007;20(3):26–29.

6. Centers for Medicare and Medicaid Services. 42 CFR Part 410 Medicare program; conditions for payment of power mobility devices, including power wheelchairs and power-operated vehicles. *Fed Reg.* 2006;71(65):17021–17030.

7. Buning ME, Schmeler MR, Crane B. Funding for wheelchairs in general. Available at: http://www.wheelchairnet.org/WCN_ProdServ/Funding/funding.html. Accessed September 25, 2006.

8. Medicare Rights Center. Forcing isolation: Medicare's "in the home" coverage standard for wheelchairs. *Care Manag J.* 2005;6(1):29–37.

9. Dicianno BE, Tovey E. Power mobility device provision: understanding Medicare guidelines and advocating for clients. *Arch Phys Med Rehabil.* 2007;88:807–816.

10. ABLEDATA. ABLEDATA informed consumer's guide to funding assistive technology. Available at: http://www.abledata.com/abledata_docs/funding.htm. Accessed November 8, 2008.

11. Ferguson-Pell M, Nicholson G, Bain D, Call E, Grady J, deVries J. The role of wheelchair seating standards in determining clinical practices and funding policy. *Assist Technol.* 2005;17:1–6.

12. Meehan R, Skolsky RJ. Navigating the options. *Rehab Manag.* 2005;18(3):34–37.

13. Guerette P, Tefft D, Furumasu J. Pediatric powered wheelchairs: results of a national survey of providers. *Asst Technol.* 2005;17:144–158.

C H A P T E R   1 1

Fitting, Training, and Dispensing the Wheelchair

The Wheelchair Fitting

Once the wheelchair is ordered and delivered by the supplier, it should be properly fitted to the patient before it is dispensed. Depending on the complexity of the order, anywhere from one to several fittings may be required before the wheelchair is acceptable and ready to go home with the patient. Evaluate (1) the wheelchair, (2) the patient's positioning in the wheelchair, and (3) the patient/caregiver's knowledge of the equipment. Make sure the wheelchair is properly configured (e.g., rear wheel axle location relative to shoulders; correct seat/back angles and seat depth) and fits well to accommodate unique postural needs, so if patients self-propel, they do it with greater efficiency. In a systematic review of adaptive equipment use in older adults (55 years or older), Kraskowsky and Finlayson found that a poor fit was the chief reason for abandoning equipment.[1]

In the end, everyone should be happy before the patient goes home with the equipment. If the final product is not acceptable, don't have the patient sign for the equipment until legitimate issues are resolved.

Evaluate the Wheelchair

- *Is the order correct?*
- *Were all items delivered?* Go through the order with the supplier and check off each item ordered to determine if it was delivered.
- *Are postural supports installed securely?* Do not place a patient into the wheelchair unless you're sure it's properly and safely secured.
- *Do all components operate (e.g., removable parts, tilt mechanism)?*
- *Do wheel locks work?*
- *Does the wheelchair fold if it's supposed to?*
- *Is the frame stable and are antitippers on the wheelchair if ordered?*
- *Are there any exposed sharp or hard edges that may cause injuries?*
- *Is the seat-to-back angle of the inserts acceptable* and set at the correct angle based on the patient's available hip flexion during the evaluation?

Evaluate Patient in the Wheelchair

First, position the patient properly in the wheelchair.

- *Are postural supports properly installed and configured based on the initial evaluation?*
- *Is the seat depth acceptable?* There should be no more than 2 inches of space between the front of the seat and the back of the knee. No pressure should exist against the back of the knee.
- *Is the seat width acceptable?* There may be up to 1 inch of space on either side of the hips.
- *Is the back height acceptable based on activity level and sitting ability?* The lower back must be supported. If the patient self-propels, the back should not interfere with UE movements.
- *Is the footplate height acceptable?* The footplate height should support the weight of the LE so the thigh is approximately parallel with the seat cushion. If footplates are adjusted too high, increased hip flexion and excessive pressure under the ischia can develop. If footplates are adjusted too low, excessive pressure under the distal posterior thigh can result.
- *In the frontal plane*, is the pelvis (anterior superior iliac spines) level, the shoulders and eyes horizontal, and nose vertical? If the patient has a fixed scoliosis, are the head and shoulders balanced over the base of support?
- *In the sagittal plane*, is the pelvis in a neutral tilt, with the shoulder and head balanced over the pelvis?
- *In the transverse place* (birds-eye view, looking down from above), are the pelvis, shoulders, and nose facing front and not rotated left or right relative to the midline? If the patient has a fixed scoliosis, is the head facing front?
- *Are rear wheels ideally positioned relative to the UEs for propulsion?* Determine whether the patient propels most efficiently when the wheel axes are aligned with or slightly in front of the patient's shoulder axes, and the elbows are in mild flexion when the patient's hands reach to the top of the handrims.
- *Is seat belt attached at the proper angle?* (typically 45 degrees)
- *If a chest harness is used*, is adequate clearance provided for the neck?
- *If a pommel is used*, is it positioned distally between the knees and not proximally into the groin?
- *If lateral trunk supports are used*, is there acceptable clearance of the axillary region with no pressure into the brachial plexus?
- *If a lap board is used*, is there sufficient space between the abdomen and the tray for clothes and respiration?
- *Is the frame stable from tipping* when the patient is in the wheelchair?

Evaluate the Equipment Knowledge of Patients, Caregiver, and Family

Does the caregiver know how to (or can the patient or does the patient know how to instruct others to):

- *Properly position the patient in the wheelchair?*
- *Operate all the components* (i.e., antitippers, wheel locks, armrests, front rigging)?
- *Fold and unfold the wheelchair?*
- *Properly and safely position straps (harness) and supports?*
- *Engage the wheel locks during transfers?*
- *Negotiate curbs, ramps, and maneuvering wheelchair?*
- *Maintain the wheelchair?*
- *Follow up?*

Training

The owner's manual is the ultimate resource for model-specific device operation and maintenance and should be given to the patient/family. The patient and family should be able to operate the new wheelchair, be it manual or power, before dispensing. If additional training is anticipated during the evaluation, the patient should be placed "on program" for training before the device is dispensed to home (e.g., training to perform wheelies). Also, ensure the following skills are learned by the patient and/or caregiver.

Using Proper Body Mechanics During Manual Patient Lifts and Transfers

Mechanical lifts are generally recommended for caregiver-assisted transfers because manual lifting carries injury risks. Nevertheless, caregivers still manually transfer and lift patients. Safety guidelines during manual lifting include keeping the load close to the lifter, maintaining a straight back, using hips and legs for lifting, using an appropriate base of support, and avoiding spine twisting movements.[2] Aside from two-person lifts, stand pivot and sliding board transfers are common.

In a study by Hess et al., who had home health aides (*n* = 16) transfer mock patients using three different single assisted methods, sliding board transfers were rated over scooting and modified stand-pivot technique as being preferred, safer, more comfortable, and performed in less time and with less force.[3] (Instrument measurement properties were not mentioned in their study.)

Proper Positioning in the Wheelchair

No wheelchair will be good if the patient is positioned poorly. In other words, first properly position the patient.

1. Engage the wheel locks on the wheelchair. This is critical during any transfer activity into or out of the wheelchair.
2. Transfer the patient safely into the wheelchair.
3. Move the patient's pelvis back into the rear of the seat until the back of their pelvis touches the back of the insert of the wheelchair. (This is not as

easy as it sounds.) Confirm that the patient's pelvis is back in the seat by gently leaning the patient's trunk forward (if possible) and then checking that there is no gap (space) between the back of the pelvis and the back insert of the wheelchair (Figure 11-1). (In some cases, a gap is intentionally created between the back of the seat and the bottom of the back insert during the fitting (i.e., "back gap")[4] to provide clearance for the patient's posterior pelvic area in order to achieve a neutral pelvic position.

4. Secure the seat belt across the patient's hips firmly (so you can fit only two fingers between the seat belt and the patient's body). The patient's pelvis must be maintained back in the seat while you secure the seat belt.

How Wheelchair Components Operate

Become familiar with how parts operate. Each company designs its components a little differently. I remember scratching my head for 10 minutes before figuring out how to remove a high-tech armrest.

- Wheel locks
- Seat belt
- Armrests
- Front rigging
- Antitippers: Caregivers should be instructed not to step on antitippers to raise the casters off the ground (i.e., for curb negotiation) because the metal tubing is thin and can easily crack (Figure 11-2). Use tipping sleeves, located on the back of the chair, instead.
- Removal of inserts
- Proper use of straps, harnesses, and positioning devices

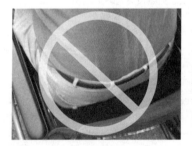
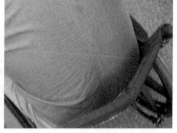

FIGURE 11-1 Positioning in a wheelchair. Confirm that the patient's pelvis is back in the seat. **(A)** Patient is not sitting back. **(B)** Pelvis is back.

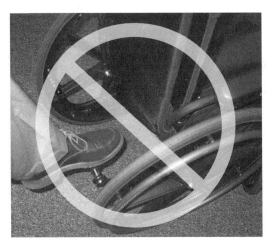

FITTING, TRAINING, AND DISPENSING THE WHEELCHAIR

How to Negotiate the Environment

Patients and caregivers need to be taught how to safely ascend and descend ramps and curbs. Some information can be found in the wheelchair's user manual. If the wheelchair must be manually lifted up or down stairs, it is critical that assisting caregivers do not lift the wheelchair from detachable or removable components, like armrests or front rigging.

How the Wheelchair Folds and Unfolds

I used to run into a family once a month who owned a wheelchair for years yet never knew it could fold. This often involves removing the inserts first. Folding a wheelchair can make it easier for a family to go on vacations. Improve their quality of life—teach the family to fold and unfold their wheelchair. Caution them, however, not to get their fingers caught between the rails while unfolding the frame.

Unfolding: Safety Precaution

When instructing to open (unfold) a wheelchair, make sure the fingers are not caught under the seat rails where they can be entrapped, and injured. Point fingers inward, toward the center of the seat upholstery, prior to exerting downward pressure on the seat rails when unfolding (opening) the chair (Figure 11-3).[5]

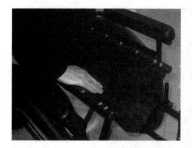 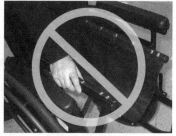

FIGURE 11-3 Unfold a wheelchair. **(A)** Point fingers toward the center of the seat. **(B)** Keep fingers away from side rails where they can get pinched.

How to Clean the Wheelchair

Most wheelchair components can be cleaned using warm water and mild soap, but because materials vary in wheelchairs, check the owner's manual.[6,7]

- *Naugahyde*—Clean with warm water and mild soap.
- *Metal parts*—Use wax with a cleaner (i.e., auto wax).
  - Avoid dripping liquid into openings of metal parts.
- *Wood, leather, and leatherette*—Use upholstery wax.
- Completely dry all components.

Wheelchair Maintenance

Have the patient/family check the wheelchair routinely for wear and tear. Wheelchair parts may loosen over time and tightening loose nuts periodically will help prevent losing parts later. Owner manuals typically include a weekly and monthly maintenance schedule and check list. If a part falls off, and it is unclear how to reinstall it, have them place it in a "wheelchair parts box" (shoebox or bag) and have the supplier or clinic reattach the part as soon as possible.

Tire Pressure Maintenance

One of the easiest ways to foster efficient propulsion is to maintain the recommended air pressure levels in the wheelchair's pneumatic tires. These pressures should be checked periodically because 50% of tire pressure loss occurs within a month's time.[8]

Dispensing and Follow-Up

Prior to dispensing the wheelchair, make sure the patient receives all supplier contact information, clinic contact information, warranty information, equipment manuals, and any special instructions including follow-up visits in writing.

Wheelchair Checkups

Wheelchair maintenance checkups may help to reduce accidents. In a randomized controlled trial (RCT), Hansen et al. found that while providing a 3-month occupational therapy–initiated home maintenance checkup, 73 of the 74 wheelchairs (that is, 99% of the chairs) inspected were found to require maintenance work.[9] The accident rate declined in an active checkup group that received the home checkup (from 5 accidents in the previous year to 0) but was unchanged in a standard care group that did not receive any checkups during the same year. (Attrition did occur in both groups during the year.) Interestingly, users were not always aware they needed wheelchair repairs, suggesting that they may not know to call for repairs if the decision were left to them.

Wheelchair Defects

If problems arise with the device that can't be resolved by the supplier and manufacturer, consult "lemon laws" in the patient's state, which may offer protection for the first year following purchases.

- Warranties and lemon laws: http://www.wheelchairnet.org/WCN_ProdServ/Funding/warranty.html
- For state by state listings, search Wheelchair Lemon Law and your state (e.g., wheelchair lemon law AND New York)
- Also see http://www.usatechguide.org

References

1. Kraskowsky LH, Finlayson M. Factors affecting older adults' use of adaptive equipment: review of the literature. *Am J Occup Ther.* 2001;55(3):303–310.
2. Batavia M. *Contraindications in Physical Rehabilitation.* St. Louis, MO: Saunders; 2006.
3. Hess JA, Kincl LD, Mandeville DS. Comparison of three single-person manual patient techniques for bed-to-wheelchair transfers. *Home Healthcare Nurse.* 2007;25(9):577–579.
4. Gilinsky G, Smith C. New wheelchair or new solution? *Rehab Manag.* 2006;19(1):34–39.
5. Hazard report: foldable wheelchairs injure patients' fingers. *Health Devices.* 2006;35(6):231–233.
6. Behrman AL. Clinical perspectives on wheelchair selection: factors in functional assessment. *J Rehabil Res Dev.* 1990;2(Supp):17–27.
7. Freney D. Pediatric seating. *Home Health Care Dealer/Supplier.* 1995;Sept/Oct:103–105.
8. Sawatzky B, Denison I. Wheeling efficiency: the effects of varying tyre pressure with children and adolescents. *Pediatr Rehabil.* 2006;9(2):122–126.
9. Hansen R, Tresse S, Gunnarsson RK. Few accidents and better maintenance with active wheelchair check-ups: a randomized controlled clinical trial. *Clin Rehabil.* 2004;18:631–639.

APPENDICES

Appendix A: Medicare's Algorithm*

Background

Mobility Assistive Equipment Coverage

CMS is extending national coverage regarding MAE for beneficiaries who have a personal mobility deficit sufficient to impair their participation in MRADLs, such as toileting, feeding, dressing, grooming, and bathing in customary locations in the home. Determining the presence of a mobility deficit will be made by an algorithmic process, as outlined in the Clinical Criteria for MAE Coverage, to provide the appropriate MAE to correct the mobility deficit.

MAE includes, but is not limited to, canes, crutches, walkers, manual wheelchairs, power wheelchairs, and scooters. CR3791 instructs Medicare carriers, DMERCs, and RHHIs to:

- Disregard the "bed- or chair-confined" criterion that has been historically used to determine if a wheelchair is reasonable and necessary as defined by the Social Security Act (Section 1862(A)(1)(a)).
- Use the algorithmic approach as outlined in the *Medicare National Coverage Determinations Manual* (Pub. 100-03, Section 280.3), Clinical Criteria for MAE Coverage (and included below) to determine coverage eligibility of MAE.

As in other cases, if data analysis indicates potentially aberrant billing, Medicare DMERCs and FIs will use these standards when performing medical review of claims.

Medicare beneficiaries may require mobility assistance for a variety of reasons and for varying durations because the etiology of the disability may be due to a congenital cause, injury, or disease. Thus, some beneficiaries experiencing temporary disability may need mobility assistance on a short-term basis, while in contrast, those living with chronic conditions or enduring disabilities will require mobility assistance on a permanent basis.

In addition, Medicare beneficiaries who depend upon mobility assistance are found in varied living situations. Some may live alone and independently while others may live with a caregiver or in a care facility. The beneficiary's environment is relevant to the determination of the appropriate form of mobility assistance that should be employed.

For many patients, a device of some sort is compensation for the mobility deficit. However, some beneficiaries experience co-morbid conditions that can impact their ability to safely use MAE independently or to successfully regain

---

* Source: Excerpt from MLN Matters: Information for Medicare Fee-For-Service Heath Care Professionals (#MM3791). Available at http://www.cms.gov. This information was gleaned from available information on the CMS Web site.

independent function even with mobility assistance. The functional limitation (as experienced by a beneficiary) depends on:

- The beneficiary's physical and psychological function;
- The availability of other support; and
- The beneficiary's living environment.

A few examples include muscular spasticity, cognitive deficits, the availability of a caregiver, and the physical layout, surfaces, and obstacles that exist in the beneficiary's living environment.

Nationally Covered Indications

Effective May 5, 2005, CMS finds that the evidence is adequate to determine that MAE is reasonable and necessary for beneficiaries who have a personal mobility deficit sufficient to impair their performance of Mobility-Related Activities of Daily Living (MRADL) such as toileting, feeding, dressing, grooming, and bathing in customary areas in the home.

Determination of the presence of a mobility deficit will be made by an algorithmic process, *Clinical Criteria for MAE Coverage*, to provide the appropriate MAE to correct the mobility deficit.

Clinical Criteria for MAE Coverage

The beneficiary, the beneficiary's family or other caregiver, or a clinician, will usually initiate the discussion and consideration of MAE use. Sequential consideration of the questions below provides clinical guidance for the coverage of equipment of appropriate type and complexity to restore the beneficiary's ability to participate in MRADLs such as toileting, feeding, dressing, grooming, and bathing in customary locations in the home. These questions correspond to the numbered decision points on the accompanying flow chart below.

1. **Does the beneficiary have a mobility limitation that significantly impairs his/her ability to participate in one or more MRADLs in the home?**
   A mobility limitation is one that:

   - Prevents the beneficiary from accomplishing the MRADLs entirely; or
   - Places the beneficiary at reasonably determined heightened risk of morbidity or mortality secondary to the attempts to participate in MRADLs; or
   - Prevents the beneficiary from completing the MRADLs within a reasonable time frame.

2. **Are there other conditions that limit the beneficiary's ability to participate in MRADLs at home?**

   - Some examples are significant impairment of cognition or judgment and/or vision.

- For these beneficiaries, the provision of MAE might not enable them to participate in MRADLs if the comorbidity prevents effective use of the wheelchair or reasonable completion of the tasks even with MAE.

3. **If these other limitations exist, can they be ameliorated or compensated sufficiently such that the additional provision of MAE will be reasonably expected to significantly improve the beneficiary's ability to perform or obtain assistance to participate in MRADLs in the home?**

   - A caregiver, for example a family member, may be compensatory, if consistently available in the beneficiary's home and willing and able to safely operate and transfer the beneficiary to and from the wheelchair and to transport the beneficiary using the wheelchair. The caregiver's need to use a wheelchair to assist the beneficiary in the MRADLs is to be considered in this determination.
   - If the amelioration or compensation requires the beneficiary's compliance with treatment, for example medications or therapy, substantive non-compliance, whether willing or involuntary, can be grounds for denial of wheelchair coverage if it results in the beneficiary continuing to have a significant limitation. It may be determined that partial compliance results in adequate amelioration or compensation for the appropriate use of MAE.

4. **Does the beneficiary or caregiver demonstrate the capability and the willingness to consistently operate the MAE safely?**

   - Safety considerations include personal risk to the beneficiary as well as risk to others.
   - The determination of safety may need to occur several times during the process as the consideration focuses on a specific device.
   - A history of unsafe behavior in other venues may be considered.

5. **Can the functional mobility deficit be sufficiently resolved by the prescription of a cane or walker?**

   - The cane or walker should be appropriately fitted to the beneficiary for this evaluation.
   - Assess the beneficiary's ability to safely use a cane or walker.

6. **Does the beneficiary's typical environment support the use of wheelchairs, including scooters/power-operated vehicles (POVs)?**

   - Determine whether the beneficiary's environment will support the use of these types of MAE.
   - Keep in mind such factors as the home's physical layout, surfaces, and obstacles, which may render MAE unusable in the beneficiary's home.

7. **Does the beneficiary have sufficient upper extremity function to propel a manual wheelchair in the home to participate in MRADLs during a typical day?**

- The manual wheelchair should be optimally configured (seating options, wheelbase, device weight, and other appropriate accessories) for this determination. Limitations of strength, endurance, range of motion, coordination, and absence or deformity in one or both upper extremities are relevant.
- A beneficiary with sufficient upper extremity function may qualify for a manual wheelchair. The appropriate type of manual wheelchair, i.e., lightweight, etc., should be determined based on the beneficiary's physical characteristics and anticipated intensity of use.
- The beneficiary's home should provide adequate access, maneuvering space, and surfaces for the operation of a manual wheelchair.
- Assess the beneficiary's ability to safely use a manual wheelchair.

  Note: If the beneficiary is unable to self-propel a manual wheelchair, and if there is a caregiver who is available, willing, and able to provide assistance, a manual wheelchair may be appropriate.

8. **Does the beneficiary have sufficient strength and postural stability to operate a POV/scooter?**

- A POV is a 3- or 4-wheeled device with tiller steering and limited seat modification capabilities. The beneficiary must be able to maintain stability and position for adequate operation.
- The beneficiary's home should provide adequate access, maneuvering space, and surfaces for the operation of a POV.
- Assess the beneficiary's ability to safely use a POV/scooter.

9. **Are the additional features provided by a power wheelchair needed to allow the beneficiary to participate in one or more MRADLs?**

- The pertinent features of a power wheelchair compared to a POV are typically control by a joystick or alternative input device, lower seat height for slide transfers, and the ability to accommodate a variety of seating needs.
- The type of wheelchair and options provided should be appropriate for the degree of the beneficiary's functional impairments.
- The beneficiary's home should provide adequate access, maneuvering space, and surfaces for the operation of a power wheelchair.
- Assess the beneficiary's ability to safely use a power wheelchair.

Note: If the beneficiary is unable to use a power wheelchair, and if there is a caregiver who is available, willing, and able to provide assistance, a manual wheelchair is appropriate. A caregiver's inability to operate a manual wheelchair can be considered in covering a power wheelchair so that the caregiver can assist the beneficiary.

Disclaimer: This article was prepared as a service to the public and is not intended to grant rights or impose obligations. This article may contain references or links to statutes, regulations, or other policy materials. The information provided is only intended to be a general summary. It is not intended to take the place of either the written law or regulations. We encourage readers to review the specific statutes, regulations, and other interpretive materials for a full and accurate statement of their contents.

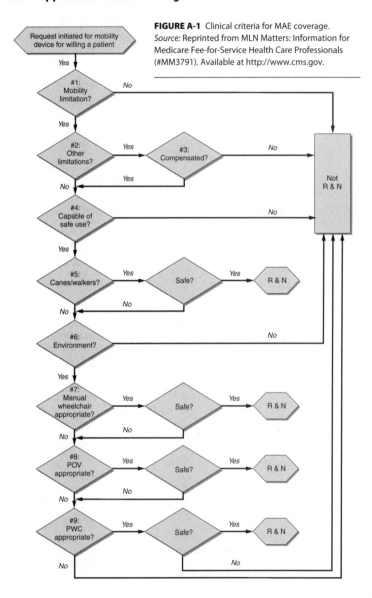

FIGURE A-1 Clinical criteria for MAE coverage. *Source:* Reprinted from MLN Matters: Information for Medicare Fee-for-Service Health Care Professionals (#MM3791). Available at http://www.cms.gov.

Appendix B: Wheelchair Evaluation Form

A form can be used to guide you during the evaluation process, remind you to assess something, or jot down findings until you write a letter of medical necessity (see Chapter 10). A form is included in Table B-1, although clinicians may prefer to design their own form. The organization follows the logical flow of the patient evaluation and captures critical information required for the prescription. Also note that this particular form emphasizes the justification of *every* wheelchair component.

Table B-1 Wheelchair Evaluation and Recommendation Form

Name_____ Date_____ DOB_____ Insur#_____ Chart#_____ Funding_____

Contacts_____

Chief complaint _____

List problems_____Successes/failures _____

Past Medical History

Age_____ Gender_____ Height_____ Weight_____

Diagnosis_____ Prognosis_____ Surgeries_____

Phys rehabilitation_____ Medication_____ Orthotics_____

Systems Review_____

Clinical Examination

Passive range of motion_____ Anthropometric measures_____ Vision_____

Skin_____ Sensation_____ Pain_____ Postural alignment_____

Active movement_____ Sitting balance_____ Primitive reflexes_____

Tone_____ Endurance_____ Strength_____ Cognition_____

Perception_____ Judgment/safety_____ Motivation for device_____

Functional Examination

Locomotion_____ Transfers_____ Sitting_____ UE function_____

Social History

Residence/accessibility_____ Level of support_____ Indoor/outdoor use_____

Table requirements_____ Travel requirements_____ Hours sitting _____

Age of existing wheelchair_____

Wheelchair Recommendation	**(What) Component**	**(Why)**
Mobility Base		
Frame size	_____	
Armrests	_____	
Wheel locks	_____	
Rear wheel tires	_____	
Handrims	_____	
Casters/tires	_____	
Front rigging	_____	

Postural Support System

        Head support _____

        Back insert _____

        Seat cushions _____

        Seat insert _____

        Trunk support _____

        Seat belt/pelvic stabilization _____

        Positioning blocks/straps _____

        Lap board _____

        Accessories/other _____

Controls _____

Appendix C: Resources and Links

Directories for Wheelchair or Seating Manufacturers

For a list of manufacturers with contact information on their wheeled mobility products (e.g., ABC wheelchair corporation), go to http://www.wheelchairnet .org/WCN_ProdServ/prodserv.html and click on Wheelchairs and Scooters.

For specific wheelchair or seating products listed by category (e.g., air flotation seat cushions) with manufacturer contact information, go to http://www .abledata.com, click on Products, and then either Seating or Wheeled Mobility.

Remaining Current with Wheelchair Information

Use a multitiered approach for staying current with the wheelchair literature:

1. Register for e-mail alerts from journals or wheelchair-related publications.
2. Conduct periodic searches for wheelchair-related literature.
3. Visit links to comprehensive assistive technology and wheelchair Web addresses.
4. Attend annual wheelchair-related expos and conferences.
5. Join local and national mobility-related organizations.
6. Participate in wheelchair-related discussion groups on the Internet.

Email Alerts from Wheelchair-Related Publications

There are several rehabilitation journals that publish much of the wheelchair-related literature. If you can sign up for an email alert on their Web site (some offer it, others don't), you will receive an email whenever the topic you requested (i.e., wheelchairs) is published in their journal. Once you are alerted by the publication, your access to that article will then depend on whether it's free or requires a subscription. If you are affiliated with a university or medical library, they may already have a subscription to that journal. Otherwise, you may be able to review the abstract on pubmed.gov and subsequently purchase the article for a fee at that same site, if you are interested.

Some journals that commonly publish wheelchair-related literature:

- *Rehab Management*: http://www.rehabpub.com.
- *Archives of Physical Medicine and Rehabilitation*: http://www.acrm.org/publications/ APMandR.cfm.
- *Assistive Technology*: http://www.resna.org/store/index.php.
- *Journal of Rehabilitation, Research and Development*: http://www.research.va.gov/ programs/rrd.cfm.
- You can also view the reference lists at the end of chapters in this book for other common wheelchair-related journal sources such as the *American Journal of Occupational Therapy*, *Disability and Rehabilitation*, and the numerous physical therapy journals (e.g., pediatrics, geriatrics).

Conduct Searches of Wheelchair-Related Literature

You can conduct a free search for wheelchair-related articles at the following links. (Once you locate an article of interest, you can acquire the article as described above.)

- *The Physiotherapy Evidence Database (PEDro)* will provide physical therapy–related wheelchair journal articles using randomized clinical trial designs or systematic reviews. Access PEDro at http://www.pedro.fhs.usyd.edu.au.
- *The Cochrane Library* provides systematic reviews on topics searched. Access the library through the Cochrane Collaboration at http://www.cochrane.org.

- *PubMed* will provide you with wheelchair-related citations within Medline's National Institutes of Health's massive database. Access PubMed at http://www.pubmed.gov or http://www.ncbi.nlm.nih.gov/sites/entrez.

    - If you are using Medline through your medical library or university, be sure to click on the box "map term to subject heading," if available, on their Web site to improve the sensitivity of your keyword search.

Assistive Technology Web Addresses

- *ABLEDATA* is sponsored by the National Institute on Disability and Rehabilitation Research and the Department of Education: http://www.abledata.com.
- *WheelchairNet*: http://www.wheelchairnet.org.

Annual Wheelchair-Related Expos/Conferences

To find annual exhibits, visit the links below. (If a link does not work, try shortening the hyperlink or alternatively, searching by name [e.g., Abilities Expo].)

- World Congress on Disabilities (WCD) Expo: http://www.wcdexpo.com
- Medtrade: http://www.medtrade.com/medtrade/show/about-the-show
- Abilities Expo: http://www.abilitiesexpo.com

Join Mobility-Related Organizations

- RESNA: http://www.resna.org
- National Registry of Rehabilitation Technology Suppliers: http://www.nrrts.org
- American Physical Therapy Association (APTA): http://www.apta.org
- American Occupational Therapy Association (AOTA): http://www.aota.org
- American Congress of Rehabilitation Medicine (ACRM): http://www.acrm.org

Participate in Wheelchair-Related Discussion Groups on the Internet

- Assistivetech.net National Public Website on Assistive Technology: http:// assistivetech.net/webresources/discussion_groups.php

Appendix D: Differential Diagnosis of Common Wheelchair Problems

We will now review common wheelchair problems you are likely to encounter.* Problems can often be solved or at least better understood by first properly positioning the patient in the wheelchair. Once the problem is identified, more than one solution often exists. For example, if the chair tips backward too easily (because of patient weight distribution in the chair), you can move the seat forward, move the rear wheels backward, or order rear antitippers. Each decision will have trade-offs that need to be weighed.

Wheelchair Is Too Small

This problem is usually seen with children because they are still growing. Much like death and taxes, growth in children is almost a given. Try to build a couple of years of growth into a seating system if patient growth is anticipated.

Possible Causes

- Patient is not properly positioned in the wheelchair (e.g., pelvis is not back far enough.)
- Patient grew.
- Patient weight gain.
- Patient wearing new brace or body jacket (i.e., taking up space in the wheelchair).
- Patient wearing thicker apparel (e.g., winter coats).
- Inserts shifted.

Wheelchair Is Difficult to Push

There are many reasons why a patient has difficulty pushing a chair. Look for problems with the wheelchair configuration (e.g., seat and rear wheel placement), wheelchair components (e.g., low tire pressure, worn parts, heavy parts), the user (e.g., impairments—weakness, pain, deconditioning, poor coordination), and the environment (hills, wind, ground conditions).

Possible Causes

- Wheel locks are locked or partially engaged.
- Wheels are rubbing against the side of the wheelchair (i.e., against the skirt guard).
- Casters are hitting the footplate.
- Footplate is dragging on the ground.
- Patient's feet are dragging.

---

* Wheelchair user manuals also have a troubleshooting section.

- Frame is bent (twisted).
- Wheel bearings are worn (may also be noisy).
- Wheel axles are not aligned.
- Wheelchair is heavy.[1]
- Push handles are too low or too high for the caregiver.
- Patient's physical disability interferes with efficient self-propulsion.
- Rear wheels are not optimally positioned (i.e., too posterior, too low) for efficient propulsion.
- Increased wheel-rolling resistance due to:

  - Low tire pressure;[1,2] flat tires
  - Increased body mass (obesity)[1]
  - Small wheel diameter[2]
  - Thicker tires[2]
  - Solid rubber tires[3]
  - Increased tire weight[2]
  - Tire treads[2]
  - Reduced floor hardness[1] (friction from floor surface, e.g., carpet, gravel, snow, sand)
  - Caster shimmy[1]
  - Toe in/toe out of wheels[1]
  - Folding frame[1]
  - Reduced maintenance[1]

- Wind[4]
- Inclines/slopes[4]

Wheelchair Tips Over (Backward)

Tipping is an obvious safety hazard.[5] Tipping problems are usually due to (1) a small base of support (frame), (2) a high center of mass (patient), or (3) a large force that pushes the center of mass beyond the base of support. Try to increase the base (frame) or lower the load (seating system) when possible.

Possible Causes

- Antitippers are not in use, not pointed down, broken, or missing.
- Patient rocks trunk or bangs head against the back of wheelchair.[6,7]
- Seating system is installed too far back on the frame.[6]
- Seating system is installed too high on frame.
- Rear wheels are installed too far forward on the frame.
- Rear wheel camber.[7]
- Wheels are unleveled, worn unequally, or missing.
- Frame is too small for the patient.
- Patient is too large for the frame.
- Patient with amputation (less anterior body mass).
- Tipping occurs while going up ramps and hills.

- Heavy bags being hung from the back of the wheelchair (e.g., backpacks).[8]
- Frame is bent.

Sliding Out of Wheelchair

Sliding generally occurs when a force (muscular or gravitational) pushes the body forward in the wheelchair. Sliding is a problem because sacral sitting may result, pressure ulcers can develop, and the patient will not be able to perform skills well when poorly supported (e.g., operating a control switch). There is also the danger that the patient can become seriously injured. A heart-stopping example is the patient whose neck gets caught in a chest harness while sliding. Physical restraint–related deaths from strangulation have been documented.[9]

Possible Causes

- Patient was not properly positioned in wheelchair.
- No seat belt.
- Seat belt is loose, broken, or not in use.
- Seat is too deep (long) for the patient (very common).
- Seat is too shallow (short) for the patient.
- Patient's hip flexion range of motion is limited (very common).
- Patient has hamstring tightness.
- Patient's been sitting too long.
- Patient wishes to get out of the wheelchair.
- Patient is in pain/discomfort from the wheelchair.
- Patient performs extreme flexion or extension leg movements.
- Extensor tone/spasticity is marked.
- Footplates are too low and not supporting feet.
- Curved seat cushion is installed backward (sloping down).
- Seat is pitched downward (front end closer to the floor).
- Recliner frame is causing increased shear force.
- Clothing is slippery (low friction coefficient).

Head Falls Forward in the Wheelchair

A forward flexed head position is a problem because the patient's environment will not be in view, feeding and school activities may be more difficult, and there is a danger of the chin covering up the air opening of a tracheotomy (if one exists). This problem is often due to poor head control. Try to address the problem with gravity-assisted support (tilting backward, reclining) rather than head and neck restraints when possible.

Possible Causes

- Head control is poor.
- Patient is tired (fatigued).

- Patient wants to keep head bent (flexed).
- Neck range of motion is limited (e.g., torticollis).
- Patient is having a seizure.
- Patient is falling asleep.
- Patient is drowsy from the effects of medication.
- Headrest is an irritant.
- Neck pain is present.
- Headrest is posted too far forward.

Trunk Leans to the Side (Listing)

It may be helpful to consider trunk listing problems as being either intentional or beyond the patient's control.

Possible Causes

- Poor trunk control (balance)
- Dizziness (vestibular)
- Perceptual disorder (e.g., pushers syndrome—in stroke patients)
- Low muscle tone (hypotonia)
- Patient wants to get out of the wheelchair.
- Patient is tired (fatigued).
- Patient is interested in a phenomenon on the floor.
- Lateral trunk support is broken, poorly positioned, or missing.
- Patient is uncomfortable sitting.
- Patient is having a seizure.
- Patient is falling asleep.
- Patient is drowsy from the effects of medication.
- Scoliosis or limited trunk mobility is present.
- Pathological reflexes are activated.

Patient Is Uncomfortable in Wheelchair

One of the primary goals of any chair is comfort. Check to make sure the patient has adequate padding to sit comfortably.

Possible Causes

- Patient is not properly positioned in the wheelchair.
- Seat cushion is worn to the base (bottomed out).
- Custom molded cushions fit poorly.
- Wheelchair parts are irritating or causing pressure.
- Discomfort is orthopedic related. (Inspect for fracture or hip dislocation.)
- Patient is sitting too long.
- Joint range of motion is inadequate to sit in the wheelchair. (Adjust seat to back angle to accommodate any limitations.)

- Patient is bony. (Consider a better pressure-reducing cushion.)
- Orthotics (braces or body jacket) are irritating the patient in the wheelchair.
- Change in medical status.

Patient "Hooks" Head Around Headrest

"Hooking" is a potentially dangerous activity. Patients may tend to lean to the side of the wheelchair and hook or move their head around to the outside part of their headrest. At that point, the patient can get stuck in that position. Stabilizing the patient's pelvis and trunk often helps to address a head hooking problem.

Possible Causes

- Patient was not properly positioned.
- Patient desires to look around the headrest.
- Poor head control.
- Poor trunk balance.
- Anterior support is not adequate and patient bends (flexes) forward at the trunk.
- Lateral trunk supports are broken, poorly positioned, or missing and patient leans trunk to the side.
- Headrest is wrong shape or not deep (long) enough.
- Neck (cervical) range of motion is excessive.
- Primitive reflexes are activated (e.g., asymmetrical tonic neck reflex).
- Patient uses headrest as a form of stimulation.
- Headrest is an irritant and patient is attempting to move away from it.
- Patient is attempting to stabilize him- or herself by using head (trying to better stabilize the pelvis and trunk).

Injuring Self in the Wheelchair

People tend to blame wheelchairs when patients get hurt. Determine if the patient's injury actually occurred from the wheelchair.

Possible Causes

- Patient is not properly positioned in the wheelchair.
- Self-abusive behavior.
- Excessive pressure from wheelchair parts.
- Hard, sharp, or moving wheelchair parts.
- Falling out of wheelchair (see the sections on sliding and tipping).
- Patient injuring self outside of wheelchair.
- Rough handling of the patient.
- Normal handling of a patient with weak bone structure (osteoporosis, osteopenia).
- Physical abuse.

Slumped Sitting in Wheelchair

The trunk may appear collapsed into flexion and patient may be sitting on the sacral area rather than over the ischia. (See also sliding out of wheelchair.)

Possible Causes

- Patient is not properly positioned in the wheelchair (very common).
- Seat is too deep (very common).
- Hip flexion range is limited (very common).
- Patient sitting duration is too long (fatigued).
- Patient has fixed posterior (backward) pelvis position.
- Patient has spinal deformity.
- Muscle tone is low.
- Back insert is spoon shaped (allowing pelvis to tilt backward).
- Back insert lacks lumbar support.
- Patient prefers a slumped position (as do I on occasion).

Wheelchair Doesn't Fold

Possible Causes

- Family was never shown how to fold wheelchair (very common).
- Seat and back inserts are permanently installed with nonremovable hardware (i.e., you will typically need to remove a seating system before the frame will fold).
- Frame is not designed to fold (e.g., rigid frame).
- Wheelchair parts interfere with folding ability.
- Frame is bent.

Wheel Locks (Brakes) Don't Work

Wheel locks must be repaired immediately if they do not operate because serious injuries can occur if they are not engaged during transfers.

Possible Causes

- Wheel locks (hardware) are loosened and not contacting rubber tire.
- Wheel locks are broken (metal bent, hardware missing).
- Pneumatic rear tires have low air pressure (see Figure 7-20).
- Rubber/tread on rear tires is worn.
- Wheel locks are working but floor is slippery (e.g., waxed floors).

References

1. Van der Woude LHV, deGroot S, Janssen TWJ. Manual wheelchairs: research and innovation in rehabilitation, sports, daily life and health. *Med Engineer & Phys.* 2006;28(9):905–915.

2. Burke ER. *Science of Cycling*. Champaign, IL: Human Kinetics Books; 1986:133.

3. Sawatzky BJ, Kim WO, Denison I. The ergonomics of different tyres and tyre pressure during wheelchair propulsion. *Ergonom.* 2004;47(14):1475–1483.

4. McLaurin CA, Brubaker CE. Biomechanics and the wheelchair. *Prosthet Orthot Int.* 1991;15:24–37.

5. Calder CJ, Kirby RL. Fatal wheelchair-related accidents in the United States. *Am J Phys Med Rehabil.* 1990;69:184–190.

6. Majaess GG, Kirby RL, Ackroyd-Stolarz SA, Charlebois PB. Influence of seat position on the static and dynamic forward and rear stability of occupied wheelchairs. *Arch Phys Med Rehabil.* 1993;74(9):977–982.

7. Cohen D. Optional but necessary. *Rehab Manag.* 2005;18(10):26, 28–29.

8. Trudel G, Kirby RL, Ackroyd-Stolarz SA, Kirland S. Effects of rear-wheel camber on wheelchair stability. *Arch Phys Med Rehabil.* 1997;78:78–81.

9. Rubin BS, Dube AH, Mitchell EK. Asphyxial deaths due to physical restraint: a case series. *Arch Fam Med.* 1993;2:405–408.

Appendix E: Body Shape

Body shape needs to be considered for a proper wheelchair fit, just as one would consider sleeve length and neck size for a proper shirt fit.

Diversity is the norm. Human beings do not all look the same. Indeed, it would be a very boring world if everyone did. When a patient does not fit well in a wheelchair, it may be because the patient's *unique body shape was not taken into consideration*. Little variations in a patient's shape can make a big difference in how the patient fits and feels in the wheelchair.

General Shape

Types of Body Shapes

People can generally be described in terms of being predominately *round, muscular*, or *fragile* (endomorphic, mesomorphic, or ectomorphic)[1] (Figure E-1).

Extreme round shapes are seen in sumo wrestlers and are characterized by round, soft, and smooth contours. Extreme muscular shapes are reminiscent of the beach bullies who kick sand in your face and are characterized by square, hard, and massive contours. Finally, fragile shapes are seen in the beach weaklings who are the recipients of the kicked beach sand; they are characterized by a thin, fragile body and delicate contours. Actually, everyone will have elements of all three body types (round, fragile, and muscular).

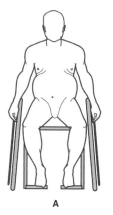
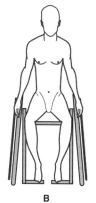
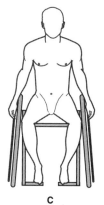

A   B   C

FIGURE E-1 Body types: **(A)** Endomorphs have round shapes; **(B)** ectomorphs have linear, fragile shapes; and **(C)** mesomorphs have muscular shapes.

When you view a patient, it may be helpful to describe their physique in these general terms. For example, a patient with tetraplegia may present with a round belly, fragile chest, and frail limbs, but a muscular neck. A patient with paraplegia may have fragile legs, but muscular arms. A third patient with obesity may have round and soft arms, legs, and trunk. No two people have the exact same body shape, so no two people will have the same fit in a wheelchair. Different body shapes will require varying amounts of wheelchair space.

Types of Body Shapes[1]

- **Endomorphic**—round
- **Mesomorphic**—muscular
- **Ectomorphic**—fragile

Age and Body Shape

Body size and proportions (i.e., relative size of body parts) change dramatically from infancy to adulthood. Children, for example, will expand with age whereas the elderly will tend to shrink. In addition, the head size of an infant is 25% of its body size whereas in an adult, head size is far less (12.5% of its body size). It is therefore important to account for the patient's age when fitting a patient to a wheelchair (Figure E-2).[2]

Infants

- Relatively large heads
- Long trunks
- Short lower limbs
- Rounded spines

Children

- Thighs and forearms will show growth.
- Spine will develop the four curves or arches.

Adolescents

Girls will begin to exhibit:

- Curvilinear shape
- Increased breast size
- Increased pelvic growth
- Greater local fat deposits

In both sexes, the lumbar arch will become more prominent.

Mature Adults

- Increased weight gain may be noted.

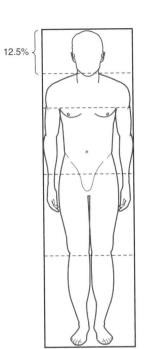

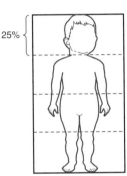

FIGURE E-2 The proportions of an adult and an infant are dissimilar.

Elderly

• Shorter trunk stature (due in part to loss of water in the vertebral disks).[2]

Gender and Body Shape

The body shape begins to show a difference between the sexes at puberty. Bone and fat distribution account for much of the shape variations between men and women, and should be considered when fitting patients to wheelchairs.

Females

In general, compared to males, females may have:

• Wider hips
• Longer trunk length
• Greater chest depth
• Shorter upper limbs (due to shorter humerus)
• Higher relative elbow height
• Shorter collar bone

- Narrower shoulder width
- Relatively shorter thighs (due to the shorter femur)
- Deeper and wider pelvis
- Wider hip position
- Shorter and narrower feet

Fatty tissue is more evident in the trunk than the limbs, with females tending to have more fat than males. Fat deposits in females may be noted at:

- Vertebral prominence (base of the neck)
- Posterior deltoid (back of the upper arms)
- Breasts
- Flanks (the sides of the trunk)
- Buttocks
- Subtrochanter (outside of the thighs)
- Abdomen (belly below the navel)

Males

Males tend to deposit fat in the abdomen *above the navel*. In addition, whereas the widest portion of the lower limb in women tends to be at the level of the subtrochanters, in men the widest area is higher, at the hip level.

Despite these differences, physical characteristics between men and women are not as clear cut as we might think. Consider each individual as falling somewhere within a continuum of having strong male and female characteristics.[3]

Weight Bearing and Body Shape

The shape of a body part will change when it presses against a firm surface. Be aware that the patient may need more seat room in the wheelchair as a result of spreading flesh (soft tissue).

Movements and Body Shape

Body parts will change shape as you move. The hamstring muscle, for example, may fit well on a seat when relaxed but may dig into the front edge of the seat due to shape changes when tensed.

Clothing and Body Shape

Clothes can affect how the patient fits in the wheelchair because clothing tends to alter the external shape of an individual. Imagine it's the 1800s and you are trying to fit a female patient in a wheelchair who insists on wearing her favorite hoop skirt undergarment (i.e., cage crinoline made of steel).[4] If patients have eccentric taste in clothing, they should wear the clothing on the day of the clinic so it can be accommodated in the wheelchair. Also note that some clothing material may possess a slippery quality (i.e., low friction coefficient), which may cause patients to slide forward on their wheelchair cushion.

Hair Styles and Body Shape

Hair can be viewed as an extension of a person's body. Hairstyle will only be a problem if the patient needs a headrest and the hair gathering behind the head interferes with contact points on the headrest. One example would be someone wearing a bouffant hairstyle of the 1960s.[4] Hats with brims will be problematic for the same reason.

Orthopedic Devices and Body Shape

Body jackets and leg braces will take up space in the patient's wheelchair. A body jacket will tend to push the patient forward and widen the patient in the wheelchair. As a result, the wheelchair seat will appear too short and narrow. Try to anticipate orthopedic device use in the wheelchair so you can plan for the additional room.

Local Body Shape: The Missing Piece in the Evaluation

Determine how much space each body part will occupy in the wheelchair (Figure E-3).

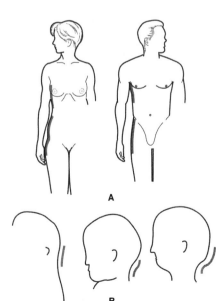

FIGURE E-3 Local body shape may differ among patients. **(A)** Body contours at the chest and hip differ between men and women and may require different amounts of seat and trunk support accommodation. **(B)** Head shape at the occipital region may vary among patients and require different amounts of occipital head support.

A

B

Head

Head shape may be predominantly large, round and spherical, cubical, or irregular in shape.

The back of the head may be curved or flat where the head and neck meet. Ears may be large or small, projected out to the side (laterally) or flat, and located at different heights on the sides of the head. In young children, ears may be more round.[2] Note the proximity of the ear to the temporomandibular joint on the side of the head.

Implications for Wheelchair

The head carries the special senses (i.e., hearing and vision) that enable individuals to interact with their surroundings. Head position also influences the distribution of muscle tonus in the extremities.[5] Wheelchair components such as *headrests* therefore may affect head position as well as muscle tonus in the body.

Neck

The neck may be predominantly short, long and wide laterally, long and slender, or apparently absent (hidden under elevated scapula).

Implications for Wheelchair

The neck provides joint mobility, muscular stability, and a passageway for oxygen, nutrients, blood, and nerve supply to the head. Wheelchair components near the neck region should not interfere with neck mobility or compress vascular, neural, or airway structures in the neck. Because of the risk of strangulation, *chest harnesses* should be used only if necessary, with adequate supervision, and at a safe distance from the patient's neck.[6]

Scapula

The scapula participates in a rhythm during arm reaching movements by gliding over the rib cage.[7] Place your right hand over your left scapula and notice how it rotates as your left arm reaches upward. If the scapula is prevented from gliding, then the individual will not attain a full reach.

Implications for Wheelchair

Wheelchair components should not interfere with scapula movements during reaching and self-propulsion.

- If a *chest harness* strap is too tightly secured over the shoulders (i.e., crossing the clavicle), it may interfere with scapula movements in patients who have functional use of their arms. This is particularly true during overhead reaching activities.

• If the back of the wheelchair is too high, it may interfere with the scapula movements associated with the recovery phase of propulsion.

Upper Limbs

The limbs may be predominantly short and tapered, massive and muscular, or long and slender.

The upper limbs serve a special role during wheeled propulsion, which can make them susceptible to repetitive strain injuries. To avoid inefficient propulsion, the correct distance of the upper limbs relative to the rear wheels should be established.

General Trunk Shapes

General trunk shape will help determine space requirements in the wheelchair.

• Chest mass may predominate over the abdomen mass.
• Abdominal mass may predominate over the chest mass.
• The chest and abdomen may be approximately equal in mass (linear).

Upper Trunk

The anterior upper trunk is characterized by varying amounts of muscle tissue and breast tissue.

• *Viewed anteriorly*, breast tissue in either sex is oriented not directly forward but rather forward and to the side.[2] The rib cage shape appears to slope downward in a medial direction due to soft tissue coverage (i.e., latissimus dorsi). In the emaciated patient, however, soft tissue is lost and the rib cage can be seen to flair out laterally and take on the appearance of a lamp shade.
• *Viewed from the side (sagitally)*, the back may appear mildly rounded (normal), flat, very rounded (kyphosis), or crooked (scoliosis).
• *Viewed from above (transversely)*, note that the sides of the trunk are rounded rather than square.

Implications for Wheelchair

The upper trunk houses and protects the vital organs (heart, lungs), permits joint mobility such as rotation, and changes volume (costal excursion) during breathing. Wheelchair components such as *lateral trunk supports* and *chest harnesses* should not be so tight against the skin that they impede costal excursion and breathing.

• If the patient (usually female) possesses large amounts of breast tissue but requires chest support, then a harness that accommodates the shape of the breast tissue may need to be considered.

- If the patient has the ability to rotate the upper trunk, then reconsider wheel-chair components that may interfere with the patient's ability to rotate (i.e., high back inserts, chest straps, chest harnesses).
- If the patient has a marked scoliosis, then a molded back insert may be needed to accommodate for spinal convexities and concavities.
- If the patient has a kyphosis (e.g., elder adult), then a curved back insert (shaped like a spoon) may be necessary to provide pressure relief for the symmetrical hump.

Pelvis

The pelvis is often the key to good positioning and the first thing one evaluates. The shape of the lower trunk (as well as the upper trunk, upper limbs, lower limbs, and head) is often determined by the position of the pelvis. The pelvis is so important, a little more time will be spent on the topic.

Shape

Viewed laterally, the low back may be mildly arched (normal, neutral), very arched (lordosis), flat, very rounded (kyphosis), or crooked (scoliosis).

Function

The pelvis is the base of support for sitting. The pelvis must act as a stable foundation for upper body activities involving the trunk, arms, and head.

The Pelvic: 3 Planes

Like a bowl, the pelvis can be moved in three different planes.[8]

1. Tilted (anteriorly or posteriorly) in the sagittal plane
2. Obliquely (elevated or depressed on one side) in the coronal plane
3. Rotated (in the transverse place)

Pelvic Positions

In the Neutral Position

- In this position, the pelvis is not excessively tilted anteriorly or posteriorly (allows for a small natural arch in the low back).
- The anterior superior iliac spines (ASIS) are level in the horizontal plane (coronal plane).
- The anterior superior iliac spines are level in the transverse plane so that one ASIS is not rotated forward more than the other one.

Posterior Pelvic Tilt (Kyphosis)
If the pelvis is tilted backward excessively, the low back will tend to round and place excessive pressure on the sacrum (increasing ulcer risk); labored breathing can ensue.

Anterior Pelvic Tilt (Lordosis)
If the pelvis is tilted excessively anteriorly, the low back may appear arched; discomfort and fatigue may ensue.

Pelvic Obliquity
If the pelvis is elevated on one side and depressed on the other side, there may be excessive pressure under the ischia of the depressed side, which can lead to a pressure ulcer.

Pelvic Rotation
If the pelvis is rotated forward on one side or rotated backward on the other side, the hips may become windswept or alternatively the individual will face off to one side rather than to the front.

Implications for Wheelchair

- Position the pelvis in neutral if possible.
- Avoid kyphotic, lordotic, pelvic obliquity, or pelvic rotational positioning if possible, as it can alter weight-bearing surfaces in the seat or affect patient orientation in the wheelchair.

Lower Limbs

Function

The lower limbs were designed for locomotion. In a wheelchair, the lower limbs can still participate in wheelchair propulsion if the feet can reach the ground.

Implications for Wheelchair

- If the patient cannot use their upper limbs well but has potential to use the lower limbs, the wheelchair frame should be low enough to the ground to permit foot-assisted propulsion. In addition, make sure there is adequate space between the back of the knee and the front of the seat to permit knee flexion during foot propulsion.
- Areas near the popliteal fossa (femoral nerve) and the fibula head (peroneal nerve) are susceptible to injury from pressure. Avoid excessive pressure from wheelchair components (e.g., brackets, seat edges, bracing) near these sites.

EXERCISE

1. **Body shape changes with weight bearing and movement.**
   Note how body shape is affected by movement, tension, compression, and respirations. Use a tape measure and record changes in width or thickness of body parts.

   a. Note how the foot changes shape and spreads out when you stand and place weight on it.
   b. Note how your thigh widens and takes up more space when you sit on a firm surface.
   c. Stand behind a friend and watch how much their buttock flesh (soft tissue) spreads in width as they sit down on a stool. Look at this phenomenon with other friends of different body types and in firm versus sling type seats.
   d. Breathing is a perfect example of how the body changes shape during movement. Notice how your chest widens in all directions and your abdomen expands forward and to the sides as you inhale.
   e. Notice how your rib cage on the right side rounds in shape as you reach to the ceiling with your right arm.

2. **The pelvic position affects how we sit.**
   Note how the position of the pelvis affects sitting by performing the following pelvic movements gently. (Only perform movements that are comfortable, without strain, and not medically contraindicated.) Sit on a stool or firm chair with your hips in 90 degrees of flexion and your feet on the floor.

   a. *First find your neutral sitting position* where you may notice a small hollow space in the small of your back. (Place your hand in the small of your back and feel it.) You should not strain. In this position, you normally place about the same amount of weight on both sides of your body. (Please note that there is much variation in how people sit. Do what's comfortable.)
   b. *Tilt your pelvis backward* by rounding the back and looking at your navel. Notice how the natural hollow area in the small of the back disappears. Notice how you tend to shorten and sit more on your backside while in this position. Also notice how much more difficult it is to inspire or reach forward from this position. (Unfortunately, this is how *many* patients sit in wheelchairs.)
   c. *Tilt your pelvis forward* by gently arching your back and looking up toward the ceiling. Notice how the natural hollow space in the small of your back becomes larger. Also notice that you would have to strain to maintain this position for a long duration.
   d. *Elevate your left pelvis* by raising your left hip up off the seat while you shift your weight over to your right side. Notice how this position

places greater weight under your right ischium and that you would become very uncomfortable if you maintained this posture over a period of time.

e. *Rotate your pelvis* by gently moving only one of your hips (left) closer to the front edge of the seat while keeping the other hip (right) stationary. Notice how this sitting position tends to twist your body to the right side so that you are no longer oriented toward the front.

As you can see, the pelvis will determine how the patient will be sitting. Ideally, you want the pelvis to be in a neutral position so the patient can sit symmetrically and function maximally. In the neutral position, there is no extreme tilting, raising, or twisting of the pelvis in any direction, a natural arch will be noted in the small of the back, and weight will be equally distributed under the ischia.

References

1. Sheldon WH. *The Varieties of Human Physique: An Introduction to Constitution Psychology.* New York: Harper & Brothers; 1940:1–9.
2. Peck SR. *Atlas of Human Anatomy for the Artist.* Oxford: Oxford University Press; 1982:215.
3. Downs JF, Bleibtreu HK. *Human Variation: An Introduction to Physical Anthropology.* Rev ed. Beverly Hills, CA: Glencoe Press; 1972:295–316.
4. Tortora PG, Eubank K. *Survey of Historic Costume: A History of Western Dress.* 2nd ed. New York: Fairchild; 1994:304–305, 424–425.
5. Fiorentino MR. *Reflex Testing Methods for Evaluating CNS Development.* 2nd ed. Springfield, IL: Charles C Thomas; 1981:13.
6. Rubin BS, Dube AH, Mitchell EK. Asphyxia deaths due to physical restraint: a case series. *Arch Fam Med.* 1993;2:405–408.
7. Cailliet R. *Shoulder Pain.* Philadelphia: FA Davis; 1991:42–46.
8. Currie DM, Hardwick K, Marburger RA, Britell CW. Wheelchair prescription and adaptive seating. In Delisa JL, Gans BM, eds. *Rehabilitation Medicine: Principles and Practice.* 2nd ed. Philadelphia: J B Lippincott; 1993:574.

INDEX